Published by
UNIVERSAL PRESS
P O BOX 37, HUNTINGDON ,CAMBRIDGESHIRE ENGLAND
TEL 0480 455456

ISBN 1-87413120 1

© John Brown . Published by Universal Press. All rights to this publication are reserved. No part of this publication may be reproduced,stored in a retrieval system or transmitted in any form or by any means, electronic,mechanical,photocopying,recording or otherwise, without prior written permission of the publishers. Whilst every care has been taken with the compilation of the publication, its content is based on information supplied to the publishers who cannot be held responsible for any errors,omissions, opinions or misrepresentation in any form.Universal Press is owned by JJLJ Worldwide.

Contents

About the Author	outside back cover
Dedication	3
About This Book	4
Introduction	6
Apple	*8*
Bread	*11*
Cereals	*15*
Coffee	*19*
Dried Fruit	*22*
Eggs	*27*
Flour	*30*
Grains	*34*
Honey	*36*
Jam	*41*
Kelp	*43*
Lemon	*45*
Lentils	*49*
Molasses	*51*
Nuts	*53*
Oil	*56*
Pasta	*59*
Pepper	*61*
Rice	*63*
Salt	*66*
Sardines	*68*
Sugar	*70*
Tea	*72*
Vinegar	*76*
Xyz	*78*
Ailments and Remedies	*81*

DEDICATION

There are many people who are in some way responsible for my becoming the person I am today and the strange thing is that many of them do not have the faintest idea of that fact!

First and foremost must rank the lease-lend nurse who was on duty at the Royal Albert Hospital in Devonport during the War and whose prompt action ensured my survival against all odds. What a lot she is responsible for!

Next must come 'Granny Orchard' who sparked my interest in all things to do with the 'magic' of Nature, and the Circus performers with whom I attempted to run away from home and who showed me a different kind of magic and made me aware of the ability and benefits of making one's illusions into realities. Also my cat 'Chuckles' who shared all my childhood dreams. Closely following behind these wonderful people came the Rag and Bone man, who had a most wonderful bubbling, hawking spit which he would produce when talking about 'him across the water'; My 'Night Princess' at Mount Pleasant, who smelled of perfume and painted her face like my 'Katy' doll; The friendly milkman who would let me ride on his horse if I asked nicely and whose rich creamy milk swooshed so wonderfully into my jug, The Toffee-apple Lady who, if I brought her my scrumped apples, would cover them with rich, glistening, delicious toffee for 1d. School mates who, in laughing at my diminutive size, transported me into the world of books, thus creating my love of learning; Tutors who had faith in my abilities, encouraging me to expand my horizons way beyond those envisaged in my wildest dreams.

To the memory of these wonderful people
I dedicate this book.

ABOUT THIS BOOK.

This little book is number two, in a series which is aimed at helping people to help themselves to health. Each little book covers different areas of our home, showing us where to find medicinal comfort from remedies prepared using the normal every day foodstuffs we each purchase from our local shops.

Book number one, dealt with Herb and Spice remedies - their medicinal qualities and use from our own 'spice racks'.
Book number two, deals with the everyday foods which we have in our Store-Cupboard or pantry.

Jennie highlights the whole food, those which have nutritional values and medicinal qualities and suggests that just by being more selective in our purchasing and use of these foods, how simple it is for us all to *Help Ourselves to Health.*

Here at last you will be taken away from the 'freakiness' attached to eating 'whole' foods and will set the record straight about the dangers of continuing to try and live healthily on an 'empty' diet, as so many of us do in this modern world of hurry and scurry, stress and convenience junk foods.

To many people, the term 'wholefoods' conjures up visions of hippies living in communes and eating nothing but nut-cutlets, or anaemic academics who spend their time discussing the relative merits of textured vegetable protein or stewed seaweed. It has also been the belief of many people, that wholefoods are only obtainable at a very inflated price from specialist outlets, needing a lot of preparation, and are often accompanied by noisy and embarrassing repercussions!

This book dispels that myth forever. Its' straightforward down to earth advice on integrating healthy, medicinal, WHOLE foods into the daily diet confirms that by taking a few steps toward healthy alternatives we don't have to make drastic changes to the Store-Cupboard.

This little fountain of knowledge, with its helpful and often very personal references and suggestions to solving some of our health problems uses the old maxim "We are what we eat". It contains a wealth of information, which, together with its' pithy humour and delightful illustrations drawn from the Author's memories, should command a place in every kitchen, containing as it does, for all ages,...

A Recipe for Good Health.

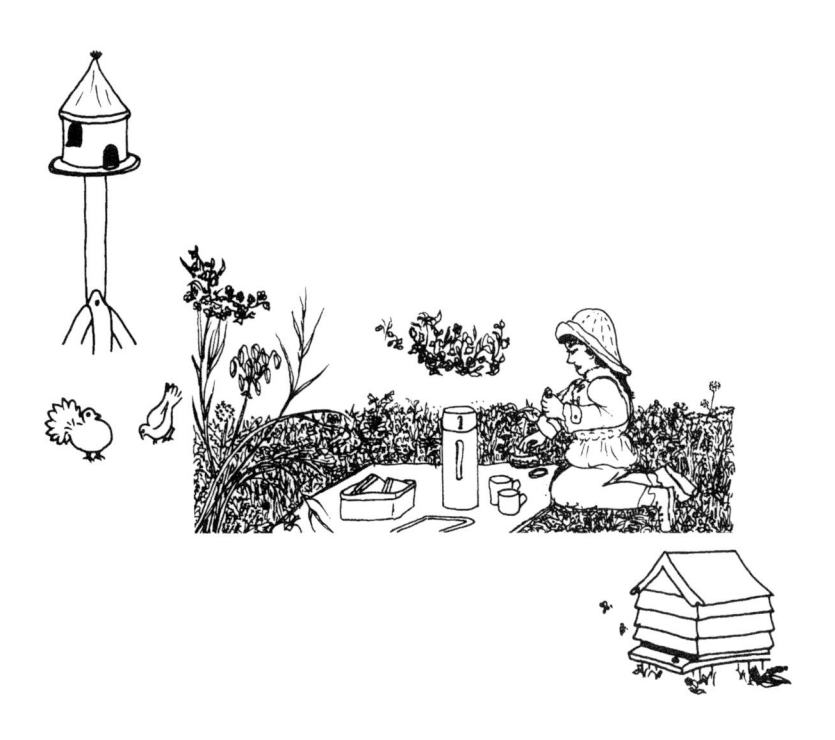

INTRODUCTION
" We are what we eat ".

How many times have we heard that said, yet how very few times do we stop to ponder the truth of it and take action which would put us on the right path to leading a healthier, happier life ? Well, now is the time for that action. Too often we purchase foods which are 'convenient', meaning that they have been chemicalised and demineralised in order to give them a longer shelf-life, increasing manufacturers profits and supplying discomfort, disease and sometimes, even death for us. Even when trying to shop sensibly and buy foods which are marked 'no artificial colourings or additives', we sometimes overlook the fact that anything with a sell-by-date of perhaps a years' time hence, CANNOT possibly contain many vitamins or minerals by the time it is finally served up on the table, therefore, without adequate supplies of these in natural form, we can suffer from stress illness and malnutrition even while appearing to eat well ! Even eating good wholesome natural foods has its drawbacks if we do not know how, or more importantly, when to or with what we should eat and drink to obtain optimum benefit from them, if this were not so there would be hardly any sick vegetarians, fruitarians, vegans or other health practitioners, correct ? To many people 'wholefoods' conjures up a picture of living on lentils, nut-roasts and soya protein in place of their usual tasty fare - unfortunately the manufacturers of some so-called 'realfoods' do nothing to dispel this myth, as it is in their best interests to promote the idea that your wholefood menu will be dull, UNLESS, you buy their tasty and nutritious products. This little book will, hopefully dispel that myth forever !

If we looked closely at the statistics of life and death in our so-called enlightened and affluent society we would be horrified to discover that the figures would probably show us the following facts:-

Out of every 1,000 deaths recorded in any period of time only 5% will have died from old age, 25% will have died violently - from road accidents, suicides, murders etc., and the remaining 70% will have died of disease! This at a time when Medical Science is using millions - even billions of pounds annually and supposedly making marvellous discoveries as to the 'cure' of illnesses which would have not occurred in the first instance, if only a fraction of that money had been spent in educating young and old alike as to the supreme importance of good nutrition. What a topsy-turvy world we live in, where men can travel in space, walk on the moon, farm under the sea, yet do not even know that there is no such thing as a common cold, but that the symptoms which are so-named, are really a plea by our over-intoxinated bodies, to give our systems a rest from the poorly balanced, un-nutritious, dangerous and death-dealing foods which we have subjected them to for so long!

Now is the time for each individual to take stock of their body and make a decision to never again put anything inside it which would cause it any form of disease either now or in the future.

Now is the time to take stock of our eating and drinking patterns resolving to start to repair the damage which has already been done and start a cellular nutrition programme for the future.

Now is the time to fill YOUR store-cupboard with food remedies turning it into a dispensary, I hope that by sharing some of my life's experiences I can help you to enjoy Good Health and Long Life.

This little book will not advise you to spend the rest of your life eating beans ..... neither will it contain a long list of all the prohibited goodies, (most of us have sense enough to know the basic facts about food as these are taught in most schools), I will instead try to lead you gently, into the path of Optimum Nutrition, by way of replacing some of the most commonly used ILL-health foods with HEALTHY alternatives which can easily be integrated into the average day-to-day diet.

What is the ideal diet? The answer is amazingly simple!

The ideal diet is one which is pleasurable to prepare and eat, gives a decided feeling of physical well-being when partaken, will give virtual immunity from periodic epidemics and viruses, gives immunity from deficiency diseases of all kinds, enabling the eater to enjoy life to the full into a fit and ripe old age. If your diet is not like this, then you could be on the way to or already experiencing ill-health through poor nutrition.... if so, take heart.. . all is not lost, by following the advice on the following pages you can gradually repair and rebuild your body, replacing each toxic NON-FOOD, with nutritious WHOLE FOODS and at the same time replacing each dying malnourished body and brain cell with a new, vibrant, supercharged health cell.

As good whole foods contain so many vitamins and minerals, once you have eliminated those de-nourishing, de-vitalised day to day habit forming foods, full of costly toxic waste, and replaced them with wholesome, healing alternatives, you will then be able to find an extensive range of remedies in YOUR store cupboard for all kinds of aches and pains and indispositions becoming Healers in Your Home. Come with me through the following pages and Eat your way to Health.

A is for Apple

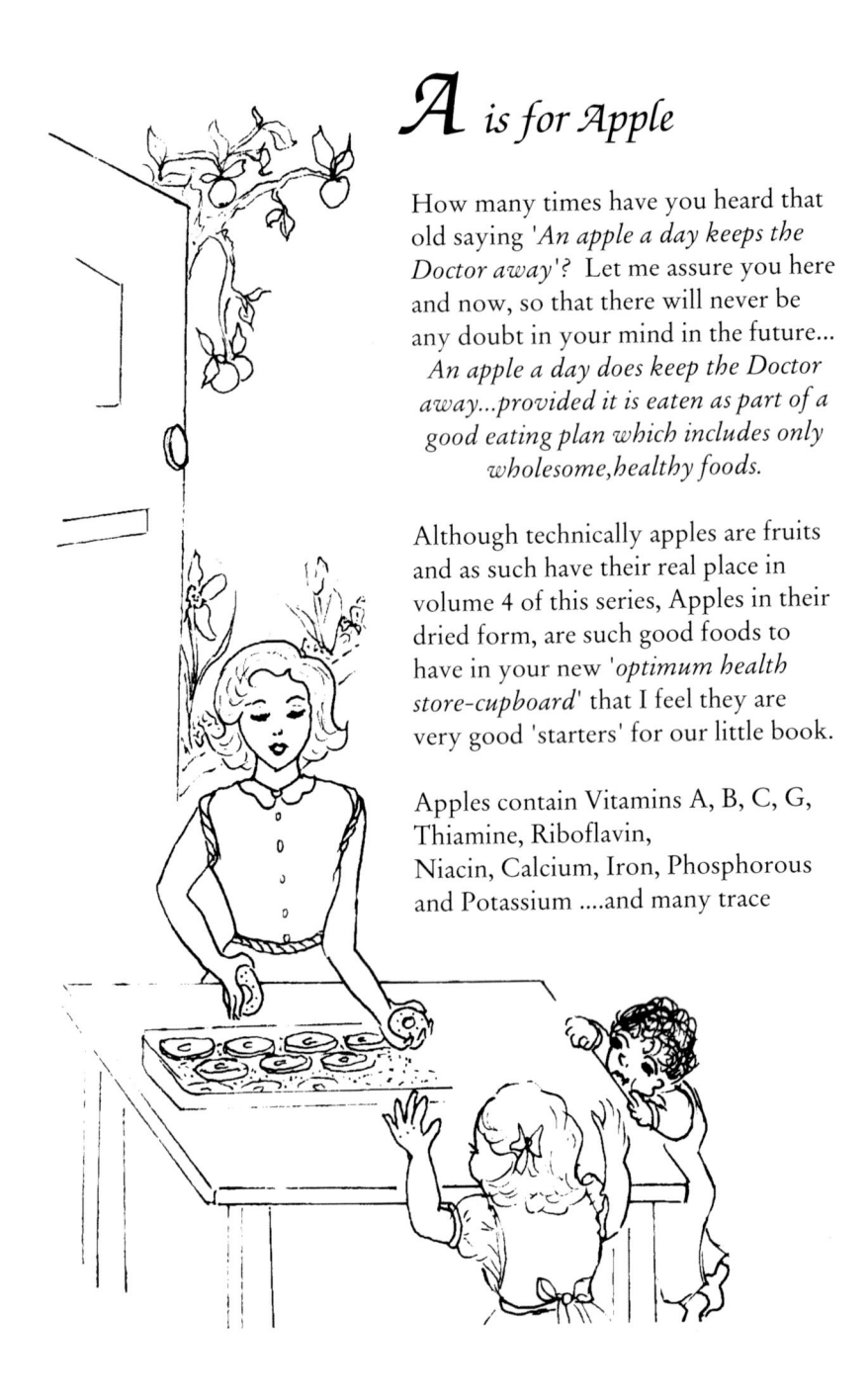

How many times have you heard that old saying *'An apple a day keeps the Doctor away'*? Let me assure you here and now, so that there will never be any doubt in your mind in the future...
An apple a day does keep the Doctor away...provided it is eaten as part of a good eating plan which includes only wholesome, healthy foods.

Although technically apples are fruits and as such have their real place in volume 4 of this series, Apples in their dried form, are such good foods to have in your new *'optimum health store-cupboard'* that I feel they are very good 'starters' for our little book.

Apples contain Vitamins A, B, C, G, Thiamine, Riboflavin, Niacin, Calcium, Iron, Phosphorous and Potassium ....and many trace elements what a wonderful health food they are!

Apples stimulate all body secretions, strengthen the blood, prevent the formation of stones and crystalline deposits, help remove noxious substances from the system and relax the nerve endings thus preventing emotional outbursts, mental and physical tension and their attendant headaches and migraine ... WOW! Just in case you are not yet convinced of the marvellousness of this wonderful food medicine, let me list for you the ailments which can be eased simply by taking an apple a day.

Anaemia, Arthritis, Asthma, Boils, Cataracts, Catarrh, Colitis, Conjunctivitis, Dandruff, Diabetes, Emotional upsets,
Energy loss, Fever, Gout, Gallstones, High blood pressure, Insomnia, Joint pains, Kidney problems, Liver & Lung problems, Muscle pain, Nail splitting, Obesity, Pyorrhea, Rheumatism, Spots, Stomach cramps, Tongue Ulceration, Urinary disorders, Vocal problems, Weight and Water retention, Worms, etc., etc., etc.!

To ensure that I always have plenty of these Health promoting foods in my store-cupboard, I keep dried apple rings, apple cider vinegar, and in case of emergencies, a pot of pureed apple-sauce always to hand on my larder shelf .... not many days of my life pass without my using at least one of them!

Often having small (and not so small) children around me with their requests for sweeties, I find the dried apple rings go down a treat... both metaphorically and literally!... I wish that more young mothers would substitute these nutritious and tasty treats, for the ill-health dealing sweets, on sale in just about every store and supermarket in the country. Giving an apple or dried apples instead of sweets, promotes strong and healthy gums and teeth they also keep the intestinal tract clean and free from worms, isn't this a wonderful health food?

In case of light injuries, bruises, cuts and grazes, stings, bites, boils and styes, simply pour boiling water over an apple ring and leave for two minutes,(or, as I used to tell my children, count to ten ten times and then shout 'apple") then remove the apple ring from the hot water and apply directly to the problem. Place and keep it there until the apple is cold, then take this poultice off the injury site, wash with the same water from the soaking and all will be left sweet, clean and germ free. This poultice is extremely effective for clearing styes and conjunctivitis and eases the inflammation in a very short time, also, a slice of fresh grilled apple works equally as well. Don't forget, if you have neither dried or fresh apples to hand, then both cider vinegar and apple puree can be heated and applied in place of them and should be in your store-cupboard.

Children will also enjoy home made Apple flapjacks much more than any commercially made cookies to take in their lunch box or indeed to have at any time when they are feeling a little bit 'peckish' and, if my children are anything to go by, this is ALL of the time!

They are simply made as follows:-

To one third of a pint (1/4ltr) of boiling water add two tablespoonful of honey and one dessertspoonful of lemon juice. Pour this mixture over half a pound (250gms) of apple rings ,which you have first separated and laid in a shallow glass or enamel baking dish and allow to stand until the liquid has been absorbed by the fruit.
Remove the soaked fruit from the dish (I find a fish slice ideal for this otherwise messy job) and lay the slices onto a bed of oatflakes in a pre-greased baking dish. Cover the slices with oatflakes, making sure not to forget the sides and middles otherwise they will go hard and chewy, and cook in a moderate oven (175c or 350f) for 20-30 minutes or until the 'cookies' are a nice golden brown. Remove each cookie carefully and leave to cool before storing in an airtight tin ... the surplus browned oats can be used as a tasty alternative to other breakfast cereals or added to meusli.. BUT.. *do not* remove the dish when children are present or you will have soon nothing to show for your efforts!

A very useful tea can be made by roasting apple slices in a moderate oven until dark brown, then storing until desired, when one slice per cup will make a very tasty tea which if taken regularly will ease the pain of Arthritis and Rheumatism and also help the insomniac to have a good nights sleep and ease all 'wamblings' in the chest or stomach. Aren't apples wonderful?

ℬ is for Bread

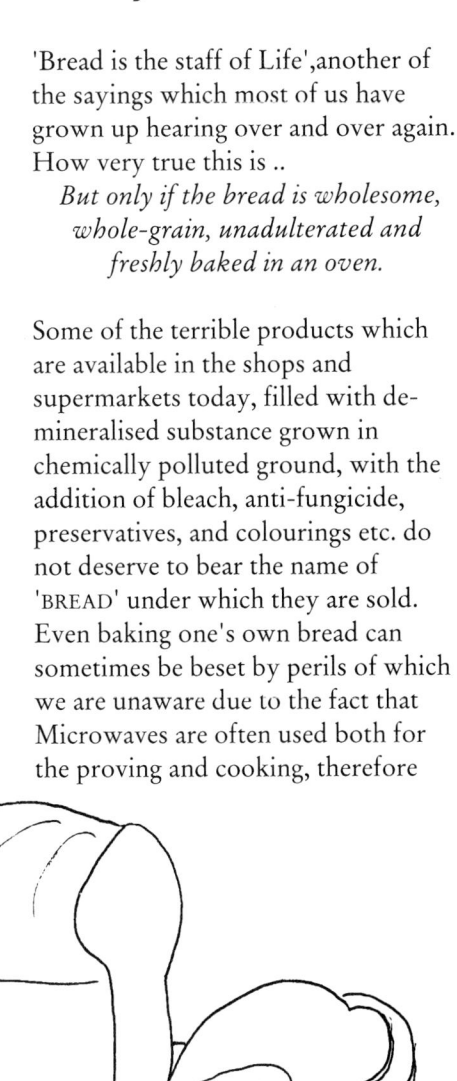

'Bread is the staff of Life', another of the sayings which most of us have grown up hearing over and over again. How very true this is ..
But only if the bread is wholesome, whole-grain, unadulterated and freshly baked in an oven.

Some of the terrible products which are available in the shops and supermarkets today, filled with de-mineralised substance grown in chemically polluted ground, with the addition of bleach, anti-fungicide, preservatives, and colourings etc. do not deserve to bear the name of 'BREAD' under which they are sold. Even baking one's own bread can sometimes be beset by perils of which we are unaware due to the fact that Microwaves are often used both for the proving and cooking, therefore destroying the enzyme action of the ingredients used and effectively de-mineralising our beautiful home-made bread and turning it into a harmful nonfood. The wheatflour which is sold in most shops and supermarkets is grown on land which has been saturated for years with chemical fertilisers and pesticides, which while ensuring that the farmer has an abundant crop with the minimum of waste, also ensures that the delicate chemical structure of the wheat is changed ...

Wheat (from which the majority of bread is made), is one of the most valuable foodstuffs know to man. It supplies us with a good supply of the essential B-Complex vitamins, Niacin, Thiamine, Riboflavin, also Calcium, Iron and Phosphorus.

Unfortunately many people are led astray by some of the wrong information given in the guise of advice, particularly
that given the case of slimming... so they fail to take advantage of this excellent and inexpensive source of health.

Organically grown, stoneground, wholemeal wheatbread, is one of the finest foods that anyone can eat and when served with nuts, pulses and other grains such as oats or rye, provides a very good source of complex protein which everyone needs, in order to live a full, rich and active life.

A lot of nonsense is put about by the meat producers of this country as to the necessity of eating enormous quantities of flesh in order to obtain enough protein for our needs, What Rubbish! All we need for a good high-protein meal is a good portion of beans on toast, a bowl of meusli or a peanut butter sandwich!

One point which I feel is very important for you to note is this ... if you cannot get 'real' bread, it is better to eat none ,than to try and supplement your diet with 'empty' substitutes. See for yourself the effect that different breads have on your internal workings.Take a slice each of any white sliced loaf and any stoneground wholemeal loaf and put each in a separate screw-top jar ,with a little warm water and shake gently for five minutes .. (this can become a good exercise for anyone needing to strengthen their wrists).... the result after only a few minutes should give you some idea of how well (or of how badly) these breads break down into flakes. The white bread as you can see has become a sticky lumpy

mess .... I for one, know which I would rather have, travelling around my internal workings and I feel sure that you will agree with me, that if you cannot feed your wonderful body with the best, then accept no substitutes!
Our bodies are the most fantastic machines that have ever been devised and, provided that we maintain them properly should give us excellent service for a long and healthy lifetime.

From childhood into old-age bread can be taken quickly, easily and in a variety of ways. One of the oldest known ways to feed it to invalids, is still the best way for a variety of maladies. Simply cut one thick slice of wholemeal bread into small cubes, put into a bowl and add hot water ... flavour with either salt and pepper if used to replace a savoury meal or a little honey if the invalid has a sweet tooth.. then, when recovery is under way, this dish can be made tastier with the addition of herbs and spices, stock-cubes, cocoa, molasses, or anything you fancy. Have you ever wondered how it was that the poorer folk in bygone days managed to survive, when by all accounts, their main staple diet seemed to be bread and vegetables? The answer is simply that, they could not afford the expensive refined white bread, so lived on the much more health-giving 'black bread' or stone-ground wholemeal and often multi-grain bread..... yes that's right... the bread which is so much in demand today by anyone who appreciates good wholesome food. Again what a topsy-turvy world!

If you have been worried that your nearest and dearest don't seem to want the so-called 'proper' meals but would much rather grab a sandwich, stop fretting, get in some tasty and nutritious fillers such as yeast-extract, peanut-butter, honey, low-sugar jams and marmalades, carob and nut spreads, vegetable pates, soft cheeses, salad vegetables etc. and let them help themselves while you relax, knowing that they are being well-fed BUT... and this is most important.. try to discourage everyone from having their bread with any of the following - Meat, Fish, Poultry, Hard Cheese or Eggs, or pastes containing any of these ... If you only remember one thing from this book, please let it be this piece of advice, your digestive system will rejuvenate.

You will no doubt wonder why on earth I should make such a statement when I promised you earlier that this book would not contain a list of 'thou shalt nots', fear not, I will keep my promise, this is one of the only two rules in this book and both are of equal importance in our journey to Superhealth. During my search for the best eating plan to restore my body to health after my ten years away from the fold of good nutrition, I studied every book, paper and thesis on nutrition that I could lay my hands on... I read from the moment I awoke... read while doing the chores... read while feeding the babies... read while in the bath... on the loo... on the bus... in the queue at the checkout... at mealtimes... even surreptitiously at church! The reason for my fascination was that I had discovered a whole new world which I had only touched briefly during my medical training... the world of enzymes and the pivotal role they play in our digestive process and ultimately our very existence.

I will not even try to explain the wonders of enzymatic action in this little book but instead condense the knowledge from about two thousand books into one vital fact which, when used properly, will enable you to revitalise your life. Honestly!

The three main enzymes which you need to know about are

PTYALIN, this is in our saliva and is activated when we chew.
This is the enzyme essential for carbohydrate digestion which will *no longer function* if HYDROCHLORIC ACID and PEPSIN are in action, as they will be immediately if any fat-containing protein foods, hits our stomachs. Thus, in order for our bodies to function at maximum efficiency remember,

You should NEVER mix CARBOHYDRATE and FAT-CONTAINING PROTEIN in the SAME MEAL.

That is the Rule.

Now EAT your way to Good Health.

C is for Cereals

Cereals are one of the most widely used non-foods in the store-cupboards of most people in this country and it constantly amazes me to hear people say how difficult it is to balance the budget with small children needing to be fed yet they are using expensive, low-energy foods such as corn and wheat flakes, bran and rice products, even oats and dried fruits which have been chemically treated, sugar coated, artificially 'vitaminised' and in fact contain very little nutrition indeed.

I remember many years ago taking part in the running of some laboratory tests during which the laboratory rats were divided into three groups, one group was fed solely on rolled oats, water and minced raw vegetables; the second was fed on packaged cereals, meat and cooked vegetables; and the third group were fed on the minced up boxes and waxed packets that the cereals were contained in together with milk and vegetables and, at the end of a six month trial period the results were most surprising....... Group one were fit, sleek, had mated and produced healthy offspring while living contentedly as a group; group three had also lived fairly gregariously, having only a few illnesses and one infant death although they did not compare favourably with group one for vitality as their coats were not as sleek and some seemed listless; however, group two, (the group which were fed on similar diet to that advocated as the most healthy and balanced, which was followed by half of the people in this country) became ill with a variety of diseases, their coats dull, eyes staring, skin and ears cankerous, tempers short, fighting, some deaths, even mothers eating their young..... Surely this must be a strong reason for changing our cereals!

What about breakfast? I hear you ask, well, what about your old breakfast? Look on the side of any cereal packet and what is the first ingredient? Corn you may say or wheat, rice, maize, or any one of a dozen good healthy ingredients... but what health can be left in a product which has been grown with toxic fertilizers, treated with nine different chemicals in the course of its growth, separated from the very germ which gives it its' essential balance of vitamins and minerals, boiled, baked, steamed, puffed, rolled, coloured, flavoured, etc., etc.?

Indeed the manufacturers know that so much of the goodness has been taken out in the processing that they have added a few man made vitamins and minerals in order to make us think that their products are now healthily balanced, well, they're wrong! What about the second ingredient? POISON... Yes that's right ... sugar... and, as the ingredients are now listed in order of amounts contained in the product, all cereals are heavily loaded with sugar, that most deadly of all non-foods and one which the cereal habit has ensured that at least half of the country is addicted to! Sometimes, as a catch for the people who are looking for healthy alternatives to the commonly known 'baddies' in the cereal field, manufacturers have added dried fruits, but these have been treated with mineral oils which can not easily be assimilated by our digestive process; or honey, but, the tiny amount of honey included cannot hope to combat the effects of the large quantities of sugar... so, be warned, and beware of cereals..... the only cereals which are good enough to feed into your fantastic bodies are those which are organic or untreated grains, simply made with no added sugar, ideally, if you cannot get these, you should accept no substitutes.

As this little book may reach you at a time when you have become well entrenched in the 'cereal habit' or you have young children who clamour for the ultra-sweet taste of proprietary cereals, even if you cannot immediately change to new health giving breakfasts ,you can change to those cereals which contain the least sugar and additives and have been produced with the minimum of processing.... the most inexpensive, readily available and most versatile of these is porridge oats. Oats are one of the best, tastiest, most nourishing foods which we have in this country and also the most under-rated. Before you start groaning about how much you hate cleaning out the pan after cooking and how much your children hate porridge... stop!... Who said anything about porridge?... Even though I personally love a bowl of piping hot porridge for my breakfast especially with a drizzle of honey on the top, having four children taught me many ways of serving oats without reverting to the 'hot glue' or ' wallpaper paste' which they hated so much and fed to the animals when my back was turned!

Children who are allowed to have cake or cookies for breakfast instead of having to sit at the table and 'have a proper meal' are much more amenable in the mornings and also the envy of their friends and, if the goodies are made with oats as their base and honey as their sweetener, mums who serve these quickie breakfast can be assured that their offspring are being fed with optimum nutrition.... what a wonderful health food is Oats!

As instant breakfast can be made by putting a heaped tablespoon of porridge oats and a little of your favourite dried fruits into a bowl, then adding hot juice and honey to taste... Tastiferous!

There are of course many good cereals on the market which are made from organically grown, whole-grains which have no added sugar, being sweetened with honey or fruit juices and which have a high vitamin and mineral content yet are very tasty.... one strange attitude which I often encounter in the course of my work is that in order for a food to be nutritious, it also has to be dull and tasteless..... nothing could be further from the truth! Next time you go shopping, look at the wide variety of breakfast cereals available in your local health food store, and, when you have decided which you will try first, taste the difference between your choice and that which you have been used to having... how does the nutty texture compare? or the fruity flavour? or maybe you prefer the chewy honey mixtures? Surprisingly, isn't the price favourable? This to my mind is one of the most important features of our new way of nutrition, it is every bit as economic, if not more so, that our old way!

If you do not live near to a health food store there are still many options open to you for improving the vitality-content of your cereals, the easiest being to only buy those products which are high in pure whole grain and low in sugar and salt... there are several on the market which are the same today as they were when they were first marketed yet enjoy quite a lot of television coverage so should be popular with impressionable children .... BUT... don't forget... Milk is a protein food, and as such should be a meal in itself... dairy foods are the toughest protein foods to digest and should not be taken in the same meal as cereals...... Cereals are best served with fruit juices, water, or on their own for optimum nutrition and that is what we are aiming for with our new health giving store cupboard.

C is for Coffee

Anyone who loves Coffee, will know how I feel when I say that since giving it up for health reasons, I sometimes dream of pots of steaming coffee being served to me and I awaken with the rich aroma still fresh in my nostrils... my one indulgence has to be that if offered coffee by my host or hostess when visiting, I do not very often refuse, (well one can't be rude can one?) however, after polluting my kidneys for several years by taking between 20-30 cups of coffee daily, and reaching the stage where I was warned about the imminent possibility of dialysis unless I changed my dietary habits drastically, there is no longer a welcome for a pot, packet or box of coffee in my store cupboard.

Coffee drinking is much more harmful to the system than tea drinking,

especially now that we have chemicalised instant coffee much more than fresh ground beans. All types of coffee contain traces of uric acid (yes, that's right, the acid which condenses and crystallises in the system, forming kidney stones, arthritis and gout to name but a few!)
As our bodies need a small amount of uric acid daily in order to function efficiently, the occasional cup of coffee will not do us any harm, BUT.. as the body always stores all the uric acid it ingests to guard against the possibility of there not being enough available at any time, *Regular intake of coffee and other uric acid containing foods is simply storing more of the same and having the effect of poisoning.* Which would you rather have... regular cups of coffee together with swelling ankles, obesity, insomnia, stress, kidney stones, gout, arthritis or some similar uric acid induced ailment? no, I opted for Health with the use of tasty alternative coffees. My larder shelf would look bereft without its' bright yellow tub of Dandelion coffee and I would feel bereft if I had to go for a long period of time without it! This wonderful product saw me through my darkest days, when I first weaned myself off my 'addictive drug' coffee.. and let me admit here and now... I was as much a 'coffee junkie' as the weakest willed drug addict and my personal opinion is that Coffee is one of the many foods, that are as deadly and as addictive as any hard core drug, the only difference is, that these food-drugs are more insidious and slower acting and no one believes how bad they really are... I do! One thing I would like to make very clear,is the very short space of time it takes, to become addicted to these food-drugs. In all my early life coffee was unheard of as my Father, Mother and Step-Father were all practitioners of the Healing Arts and did not allow the family to eat or drink anything which would harm the Living Temples of their bodies.. I did not start drinking coffee or taking non-foods into my body until my marriage and settlement on an estate full of young families who introduced me into the 'coffee morning and sherry evening set'. ONLY TEN YEARS LATER I WAS A MENTAL AND PHYSICAL WRECK! This can be verified by my medical records, which show that the first time that I ever consulted a G.P. was when I became pregnant with my first baby....Ten years, eight pregnancies, one nervous breakdown, and umpteen 'secondary' illnesses later, such as kidney, circulation and spinal problems, as a daily outpatient at the hospital with a home-help to do my housework, taking ten different types of medication daily... I had become what I ate and drank... POISON..
I thank God daily that at that point, I saw the light, returning to the eating

patterns of my youth and saving my own life!
One of the very first poison-foods which was eliminated from my store-cupboard on my long haul back to health was of course my then mainstay ... coffee! Coffee is often used in medicine as a nerve stimulant... for which it is excellent BUT ONLY IN SMALL DOSES! Imagine the effect on the body, if the nerves are in a constant state of stimulation and never rest... the result is TENSION, one of the many complaints of the so-called 'civilised' world today (Hardly surprising as the most 'civilised' drink is, coffee).

On the other hand, one of the most nerve-relaxant and health giving drinks available on the market today and one which is readily available in instant powder or granulated form is, Dandelion Coffee. Containing as it does Vitamins A, B, and C, Thiamine, Riboflavin, Niacin, Calcium, Iron, Phosphorous and a host of the trace elements essential to good health, it is a veritable 'medicine- chest' on its' own and so simple to use!

Let me just list for your some of the many ailments it will bring relief for ... ready?... How about these...
Anaemia, acidosis, anorexia, arthritis, bronchitis, blood pressure, (both high and low as it is a regulator), circulation problems, colds,constipation, catarrh, diabetes, emaciation, eczema, gallstones, gonorrhea, insomnia, kidney ailments, liver ailments, obesity, rheumatism, spots, spleen-fever, syphilis, toxaemia, verruca, warts, whitlows and worms! What a Healthfood indeed! If you have Coffee on your larder shelf and drink more than an occasional cup, then the best thing you can do to Help yourself to better health, is to throw it out and replace with a tin, box or jar of wonderful deep- cleansing, health-giving and gently stimulating, Dandelion Coffee, then drink yourself healthy.

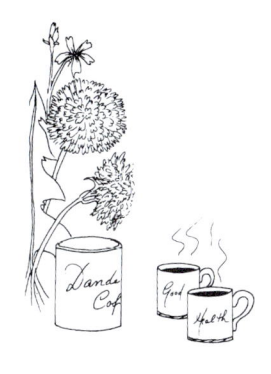

$\mathcal{D}$ is for Dried fruit

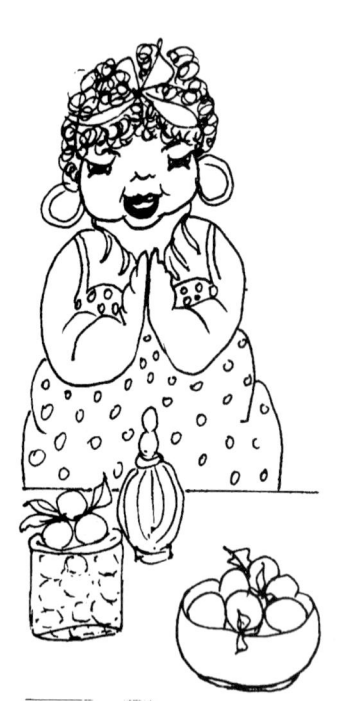

Almost everyone has the odd packet of dried fruit in their store-cupboard, but how many of you realise just how jam-packed with nutrition they are? Containing as they do a variety of the B vitamins together with A and C, calcium, phosphorus, iron and potassium, is it any wonder that children, who are so much more instinctive in their habits than adults, would often rather grab a handful of dried apricots or raisins, than stop their play to sit and have a 'proper' meal!

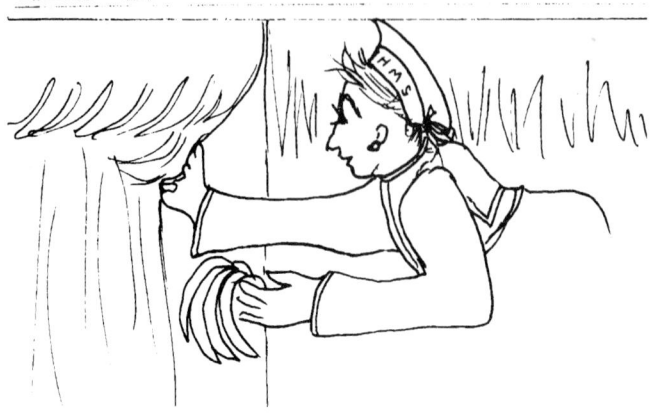

I always feel that it is a great shame that modern cookbooks do not contain the recipes for the wonderful concoctions, which my great-aunt Boadicea used to concoct for her many great-nieces and nephews when they visited her at the weekends, and nowhere in the world have I yet met a dish to equal my aunt Mollie's Raisin-custard-cups... how we loved to visit these very wise ladies, who never made us eat 'sensible' food but instead gave us strength-building foods disguised as 'special treats'.

During and just after the war years when fresh citrus fruits were all but unobtainable, we were kept in good health and spirits with our aunts' carefully hoarded dried fruits, of which the favourite was undoubtedly the dried apricots, which one of our uncles obtained 'under the counter' on the 'Black Market",which conjured up deliciously frightening visions of exotic places,with enormous turbanned stallkeepers with our favourite uncle sneaking behind their backs and crouching down in under the stalls to get some of our favourite goodies for us! How fortunate we are to be able to obtain them so inexpensively and easily today, as a food they are worth their weight in gold.

My Grandmama always soaked her dried fruit in boiling water overnight, then before using the fruit for cooking, she would strain off the juice and bottle it and keep it on her cool-shelf in the larder, to administer it in spoonful doses before we went to bed ,to ensure that we 'kept regular' as she so delicately put it. Surely a more pleasant way of guarding against constipation than taking laxatives, as so many people have to today. I can also remember this juice being very soothing, when I had a cough or sore throat, particularly that dry tickly sore throat which keeps children awake at night. If you have irregular or tickly children, use your fruit soak.

Another very tasty treat which one of my many aunts used to give to me when I was 'under the weather', was current-balls. She used to let me make them for myself by mashing currant's into a paste with a fork and adding a few grated 'monkey nuts', which if I was very careful, I could grate on the nutmeg grater and if I was very tearful, there would be a tiny sprinkle of cinnamon or nutmeg added too... How I used to love rolling the mixture into equal-sized balls and licking my fingers afterwards, and how quickly the restorative properties of the currant's and spices soothed and healed and lifted my spirits. Try this the next time you have a child who seems to be low in energy, yet does not have a specific complaint, it works wonders.

Nowadays when dried fruits and nuts are plentiful, these currant-balls are much tastier if mixed with and rolled in grated coconut which, as well as all the vitamins and minerals found in the fruit, also contains Iodine, which is a very valuable mineral for growing children, when in its natural form and an invaluable 'nibble' for anyone trying to lose weight!

One problem which seemed to be rife just after the war was Worms.... not the common or garden sort but embarrassing, secret, itchy, intestinal worms and any child known to have them was fed with dreadful saccharine covered chocolate coloured horrible tasting worm cakes... they were also teased unmercifully, by those of us who did not suffer from this complaint, and, thanks again to my Grandmama, I was one of the latter (although, had she known the part I played in the teasing, a certain part of my anatomy would have soon needed a remedy to soothe stings!) Be that as it may, with so many children having and playing in close proximity to cats and dogs nowadays, it is hardly surprising that worms once again, are a part of their lives and in order to make your child's' medicine as pleasant as possible to take, go to your store-cupboard for a remedy. For intestinal worms, toxaemia, skin pimples and all other blood impurities, simply either give the sufferer three dried apricots to eat every night last thing before going to bed, or soak some apricots overnight (which you intend to use next day for baking), in enough boiling water to cover them and give the sufferer three tablespoonful of the juice first thing in the morning on an empty stomach. A foolproof and tasty medicine.

One highly concentrated and most nourishing dried fruit food and one which is invaluable for people suffering with poor digestion, stomach ulcers, colitis, pyorrhea, anaemia and piles to name but a few, is the much overlooked and under rated Date! One of the richest foods in natural healthy carbohydrates and *not* acid-forming, a few dates make an excellent substitute for a full meal, they are especially good for nursing mothers, when their high vitamin and mineral content feeds mother and baby too!

As no chapter on dried fruit would be complete without at least one piece of advice regarding the much maligned Prune... let me make one very important and often overlooked point about prunes. *Prunes should be eaten dried or soaked. But never, never boiled!* As well as their very high vitamin and mineral content which have given prunes their well deserved reputation as a remedy for anaemia, constipation and haemorrhoids, they also contain a high concentration of oxalic acid which, when boiled, leaches the calcium content from the body! NEVER BOIL YOUR PRUNES! One delicious way of taking prunes, is to take one cupful of prunes which have been soaked overnight, stone and mash together with one cupful of crumbled digestive biscuits, one cupful of desiccated coconut and enough clear honey to bind the mixture into the texture of pastry... roll into balls, then flatten into cookies on a tray covered with coconut or crushed nuts and refrigerate until needed.... or hide them if you have children! Cookies to increase vitality and blood circulation! These cookies are especially useful as a 'special treat' for an invalid who does not feel hungry, yet needs to take in some energy foods.... try them topped with fresh cream or ice cream! A quick pick-me-up and popular with young and old alike, is the Prune and Peanut butter sandwich. This is simply made by using Peanut butter instead of butter, spread on wholemeal bread, then spread with drained, soaked prunes. If anyone has a sore throat substitute honey for peanut butter. This also makes a quick and tasty dessert if warmed under the grill until golden brown and slightly crisp and serve with piping hot custard. If on the other hand, a cold sweet is preferred such as in the case of tonsillitis, whip sieved prunes into ice-cream....mm.... delicious!

Figs are another dried fruit which often get overlooked except for the little packs that find their way into most homes at Christmas time. What a shame this is. Figs are one of the few foods which are richer in nutrients after being sun-dried than they are when fresh....they are also cheaper to buy in this form! Again the A. B. and C. vitamins with Calcium, Iron and Phosphorus with many trace elements are very much in evidence in the fig, hence its usefulness in cases of Anaemia, asthma, abscesses, boils, circulatory problems such as Raynauds disease, coughs, colitis, constipation, diverticulitis, emaciation, gout, low blood pressure, pleurisy, quinsy, rheumatism, skin diseases, sore throats, tuberculosis and ulcers in the digestive system. Children and old people particularly, will feel the benefit of including figs in their diet as often as possible, as their mineral content is at least three times as high as that of most fresh foods... they are very quickly assimilated by the body...they need no preparation... their only drawback is the pips! Of course the fig really comes into its own when boiled and the juice used as a laxative. How well I remember being given my 'daily dose' as a tot, I must have been one of the most regular children for miles around! This syrup was also given to anyone having a sore throat, cough or 'tummy-ache' and always seemed to bring fast relief. (I think the most attractive thing about having this syrup of figs was the knowledge that we were due for a treat next day for tea ... Stewed figs, drizzled over with clear honey and topped with a swirl of fresh clotted cream!)

Hot stewed figs, when slit open and applied to an inflamed boil or abscess or sore gum, makes an excellent drawing poultice, which leaves the injury site clean and germ free.

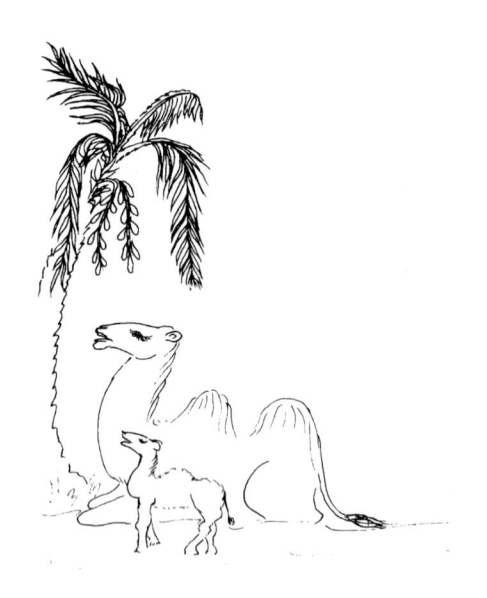

$\mathcal{E}$ is for Eggs

Although eggs are mostly stored in the refrigerator, and will have a mention in book five of this series, they should ideally be bought fresh daily and kept at room temperature in order to get the maximum nutrition from then. I keep mine in a rack, all neatly placed with their narrow end downwards on the cool shelf in my store-cupboard, so this book is the place for them!

The egg is another of Nature's miracle foods, a complete food in itself, high in protein, easily digestible and each one containing twice as much lecithin, which the body needs, in order to burn off the amount of cholesterol it contains, what a health food! Eggs again are under rated and much maligned, if given their correct place in our diets. Eggs are a storehouse of vitamins and minerals, and contain

vitamins A. B. B6. B12. D. E. Thiamine, Riboflavin, Nicotinic acid, Pantothenic acid, Folic acid, Biotin, Calcium, Iron, Zinc in balanced quantities as well as many trace elements which, although in minute amounts, act as does the tiny amount of yeast we use when baking bread.... they make it right!
I have a very dear *young* friend who at 50 years of age, only looked and acted as if he was half of that age. Having twice walked around the world, taking nothing with him but a spare pair of plimsoles and a toothbrush and who swore to me that his only foods were honey, fruits, nuts, berries and an egg a day. He is now approaching 80 and has recently walked along the course of the River Ganges in India and is contemplating a trot around the Himalayas... *This youngster* really does go to work on an egg! Recently the egg has been made to appear the villain for the role it plays in cases of heart attacks, high-blood pressure, strokes etc., and many 'slimming' organisations, recommend their members to restrict their egg intake to one or two a week... What a shame it is, that they do not instead advise their members to replace their meat in their diet, with a lightly cooked, low calorie, energy giving, nutritious, inexpensive egg, and make sure that each meal is preceded and followed by a glass of water. Thus making sure that no residues remain in the system to 'clog up the works', while we USE the eggs' nutrients.

Most of the troubles attributed to eggs, really have their base in the fact, that because our diets are so high in chemicals, AND, because we do not allow our bodies time to digest a meal before overloading them with another one, AND, because we mix the wrong foods together when having so called 'balanced meals', our bodies never have time to utilise,the eggs' wonderful nutrients. They simply ferment, causing gluttony-induced problems which medical science with all its wisdom, blames not on us the real culprits, but throws back on to the innocent victim.... the egg! However, in order for the egg to function at its best as a health food,and I'm going to surprise you now, so don't forget, *EGGS ARE NOT COMPATIBLE WITH WHEAT.*
Invalids needing a light and nutritious meal, children who have been ill and off their food, even tired mums who need a pick-me-up,will all greatly benefit from having a dish of home-made egg-custard. Which is simply made by whisking six eggs into a pint of milk, sweetened with honey, sprinkled with nutmeg and cooked on 350f. or 175C for an hour... BUT... much of the goodness is lost if it is cased in pastry or served with bread

Eggs have been used in medicine for thousands of years both internally to strengthen the system and externally to heal. The most well know being that of a very good remedy for nappy-rash in infants. Although the widespread use of disposable nappies has done a lot to keep little bottoms comfortable, sometimes, most often during teething, and especially in hot weather, rashes start to appear, often accompanied by tension and stress for Mum. The next time this happens to you, simply separate out the white of an egg, whisk until it 'peaks' and apply liberally to the affected parts.... soothing for mum and baby alike, magic! This is also a very good remedy for bedsores. I can remember my aunt applying it to my cousin who was bedbound for a long time, using a feather to apply the potion to the tender places. No need to waste the egg yolk though just add one tablespoonful of either fine ground oatmeal, stoneground wholemeal flour, kelp, powdered brewers yeast or wheatgerm and a teaspoonful of clear honey, mix to a smooth paste and apply to the face as a quick, soothing masque at the end of the day. I personally apply this while running my bath and keep it on all through my bath, so that all the nutrients have plenty of time to work, then wash off with tepid water about twenty minutes later. This leaves my skin clear, taut and shining with good health, and as soft as the proverbial baby's bottom, is that how the saying originated? For rejuvenating skin which has become like parchment either through age, or more likely, inadequate nutrition, simply beat the egg yolk together with an equal amount of corn or olive oil, apply to the skin and lie down comfortably with your feet slightly higher than your head for about half an hour, wash off with tepid water, then marvel at the wonders of adding an egg!

$\mathcal{F}$ is for Flour

All of us use flour of one kind or another for baking in the home yet how many realise that simply by changing the type of flour we use we can help ourselves to better health? It's true! Just as it is most important that our daily bread be only of the very best quality possible to provide us with optimum nutrition, so too the importance applies to our flour.
There are many flours available on the market today as more and more of our supermarket merchandisers realise that we are no longer satisfied with inferior or polluted foods and, unlike the 'dark ages' when I was clawing my way back to health, good wholesome flours are readily and inexpensively available in most large stores and supermarkets anywhere in the county. Wheatflour, stoneground and wholemeal is available both in plain and self-raising

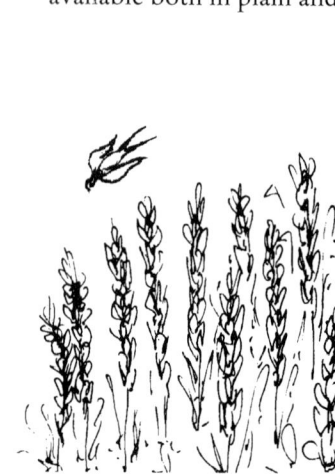

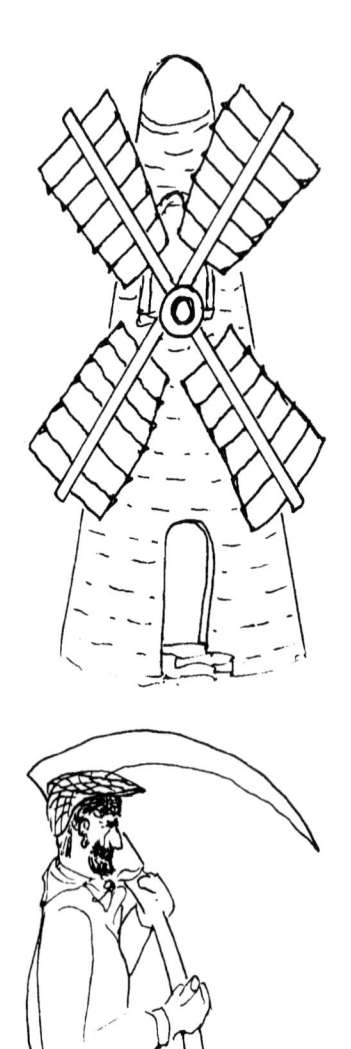

and should replace the de-naturised, chemically treated and bleached white flour in your store-cupboard immediately... once you have got used to its pleasantly nutty taste you will wonder why you ever used non-flour. Being especially rich in the B-Complex vitamins, wheatflour and the goodies made with it bring especial benefits to young children, nursing mothers, sufferers of physical and mental stress, and particularly people suffering from 'sluggish bowel'. Using 'real flour' has the added advantage that all sorts of cookies can be made with it for young children to grab when they 'have no time' for a meal, and they will be having just as much (if not more) nutrition than they would have had from the traditional meat and two veg! Get yourself some today!

Oatflour is a very special flour which is becoming more readily available, yet in some localities it is still only available in Health food stores... however, if you persist and keep on
asking at your supermarket you may find as I did that it suddenly appears on the shelves. It is usually packed in small amounts so, in the unlikely event of anyone finding it not to their taste, it can soon be used up for cosmetic purposes and there will no waste. Personally I like it more than the wheatflour as there seems to be more 'body' in oatmeal bread, muffins etc.

Oatflour, as wheatflour contains many of the B-Complex vitamins also vitamin E. Calcium, iron and phosphorus in appreciable amounts, but, unlike other grain-plants, Oats have resisted all of Mans' efforts to change its' delicate chemical balance so it is a totally natural, unadulterated, unpolluted Health Food.

Do make sure that you get wholemeal oatflour as this has the so important oatbran in it which is invaluable for not only regulating the bowel but also for stabilising blood sugar. This is a very valuable food for diabetics, hypoglycaemics and for anyone who as a tendency to get irritable if they go for too long without a meal. As oatmeal has for centuries been used as a general body builder and muscle developer, helping the heart and glands to function at optimum efficiency and visibly improving the condition of skin, hair, teeth and nails within a very short time of its integration into the daily diet, I do not need to say much more about it to persuade you to include it in your next shopping list do I? Good for you, Well done!

Rice Flour is another handy flour to add to the optimum nutrition foods in your store-cupboard as it is a convenience food with none of the drawbacks of the so-called convenience foods available on the market at present.

Not only containing many B-Complex vitamins together with Vitamin B6, Vitamin K, Calcium, Iron, phosphorus and potassium, Rice flour is an easily digested food which, as it contains all of the necessary carbohydrate requirements, is an extremely valuable recovery food for anyone who has suffered a long or debilitating illness and who has little appetite. Being useful as a quick and sure remedy for diarrhoea was enough to ensure its place on my larder shelf and many a nasty bout has been 'nipped in the bud' by simply adding a little cold water to a dessertspoonful of rice flour, mixing it to a creamy consistency and getting the sufferer to swallow down quickly ... with small children this is better if flavoured with a smidgen of honey! Anyone suffering from Colitis, stomach ulcers or any intestinal complaints where food must be very bland in order to avoid complications after eating, will benefit greatly from having their baking done with rice flour instead of grain-flours as the texture of riceflour is as fine as Cornflour, (Cornflour incidentally is another fine cure for Diarrhoea if used in the same way as Rice flour, adding a little cinnamon) and there will be no 'bits' in the food to cause irritation of the internals! As an 'instant' breakfast, a little riceflour mixed to a paste with hot water and drizzled over with clear honey can be a boon to busy mums, flavouring with yeast extract makes instant soup!

Potato flour is another very good stand-by to have in your new health food store cupboard, and, as it is such a rich source of Vitamins A, B-Complex, C, Calcium, iron, phosphorus and potassium plus a host of trace elements,it is one which should be made use of as much as possible. Having this flour readily to hand gives you a whole new range of 'fillers' for family meals without having to resort to 'potatoes with everything' as seems to be the modern mealtime habit... Pancakes, pizza, muffins, flapjacks etc. all sound like naughty and delicious 'junk' food and as such are welcomed by young people where 'proper' meals are often scorned... so .... give them what they want, BUT, use potato flour to make them with. They are not only tasty but GOOD! Potato muffins, made in just the same way as ordinary muffins, buns or fairy cakes are made, but substituting potato flour for the ordinary flour, honey for the sugar, and adding a pinch of nutmeg to the mixture, makes a delicious and different supper dish, which is easy on the digestion and encourages sound sleep. Potato flour is also a good standby to have in case of stings and bites as, a little flour mixed to a paste with warm water and pasted on the sting, will draw the poison out as it dries. As potato flour is also rich in organic salts and has powerful alkalizing effects on the system, a nourishing, tasty and very easily digestible quick soup can be made, by mixing one heaped tablespoonful of potato flour with enough cold water to form a paste, then adding boiling water, stirring continuously until the required thickness is obtained, flavour with herbs etc, and simmer for a few minutes to enrich the flavour... delicious!

There are of course many other flours available which you may like to experiment with, Barley, bean, buckwheat, corn, maize, nut and rye flours to name but a few, and most of them contain very similar properties, PROVIDED that, you ensure that they are of the best possible quality, fresh, unadulterated with additives, preservatives, and colourings etc.. Experiment with your cooking and baking and help yourself to health at the same time.

I must make a special point about Buckwheat flour as this contains appreciable amounts of Rutin, an essential element to help heal and strengthen tired, worn and damaged tissues, veins and capillaries anywhere in the body, improving their tone and texture and thus enabling the body to deal more efficiently with its movement of water within the bloodstream, particularly between the tissues. This helps the circulation and brings relief to sufferers of many problems involving tissue weakness and/or fluid retention, particularly Raynaud's phenomena, weak and broken capillaries, varicose veins and ulcers, intermittent claudication, 'restless legs' and oedema. If you suffer from any of the above complaints try adding buckwheat flour to your cooking and treat yourself to helpings of health.

Buckwheat flour can also be used as a soothing ointment for bruises, varicose or itching veins, and haemorrhoids, simply by adding a little cold water to the flour and mixing to a stiff paste, then applying to the affected parts as needed. The addition of a teaspoonful each of lemon juice and honey to the above makes a cream to banish broken facial capillaries.

G is for Grains

Grains are a very essential part of our diets and, should be eaten every day in one form or another, but as I have covered their properties fairly comprehensively in the chapters on Bread and Flour, I will not bore you by repeating myself, instead I will share with you a few important and not widely know facts about grains. This heading includes barley, corn, oats, rye, maize and wheat. One specific point about them which I feel it is very important for you to remember, is the fact that GRAINS ARE NOT COMPATIBLE WITH:-

MEAT, FISH, POULTRY, EGGS OR HARD CHEESE

If you forget everything else I have written, please, for your health's sake, never forget this fact. Once the Hydrochloric acid in the digestive system has been activated in order to digest the first class protein foods such as those listed in capitals above, the Ptyalin necessary for the digestion of starches contained in grains, ceases activation until every trace of protein is digested and, as this can take anything from four hours in a healthy system, and up to seventy two hours, in a very sluggish or run-down system, you can imagine what must be happening to the half-digested starches in the system while they are waiting around in the hot moist conditions of the intestine. That's right... they ferment! Fermenting grains cause massive releases of gas, distention, discomfort and drowsiness, and can cause ulcers, colitis, irritable bowel, gastritis and other painful complaints such as diverticulitis. No wonder the old folk used to say 'don't get your bowels in a ferment'... it's painful!

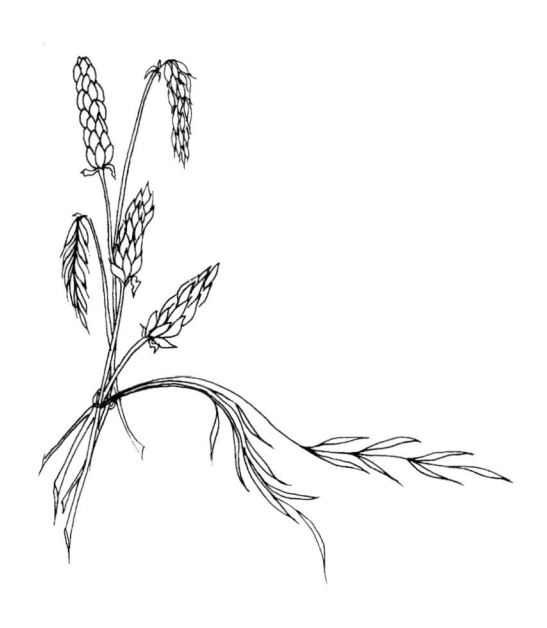

$\mathcal{H}$ is for Honey

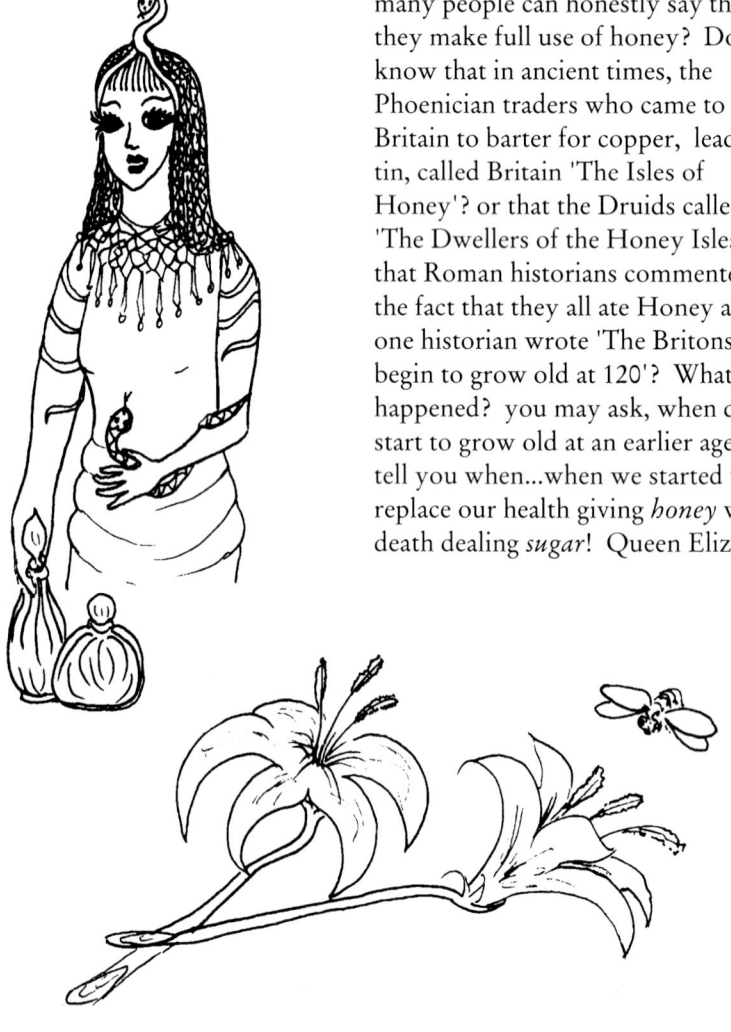

Honey.... Nectar of the Gods, Food of Love, Medicine of the Soul, valued all over the world for thousands of years and quite rightly so, as the greatest gift ever given to man. Yet again, how many people can honestly say that they make full use of honey? Do you know that in ancient times, the Phoenician traders who came to Britain to barter for copper, lead and tin, called Britain 'The Isles of Honey'? or that the Druids called us 'The Dwellers of the Honey Isles'? or that Roman historians commented on the fact that they all ate Honey and, as one historian wrote 'The Britons only begin to grow old at 120'? What happened? you may ask, when did we start to grow old at an earlier age? I'll tell you when...when we started to replace our health giving *honey* with death dealing *sugar*! Queen Elizabeth the First, started the rot (quite literally), when she developed a craving for sugar cane which was called The Honey-Bearing Reed and gorged herself on it to such an extent, that her teeth rotted and blackened and her hair dropped out! She would not have been a very good advertisement for the sugar producers of today, who are still trying to persuade us that their produce is good for us! Had the Lady kept true to her Heritage and continued to eat Honey in large quantities, I have no doubt that she would have gone to meet her maker, with fine healthy teeth and a full head of that lustrous red hair, for which she was so famous and lauded about in her youth! Be sure that you ALWAYS have Honey in your store-cupboard.

If all of the scientists in the world got together and pooled all their knowledge, THEY COULDN'T PRODUCE A POT OF PURE HONEY This is not a fairy tale ......I kid you not... Nature wins once more! Magical, Marvellous Honey, everlasting by
its nature (Honey which was sealed into the tombs of the Pharoahs of Egypt over 3,000 years ago, has been found by modern archaeologist in perfect condition and still tasting delicious!) Honey cannot contain any insecticide or pesticide residues, however polluted the land may be, where the bees gather their nectar, as bees have no resistance to chemicals and would die almost immediately on coming into contact with them, thus ensuring that no pollution is taken back to the hive and that the honey made is always pure.

OF ALL THE FOODS AND MEDICINES IN THE WORLD,
HONEY IS THE BEST

The United States Bureau of Entomology in Washington confirm that if placed in Honey, dysentery-causing germs die within 48 hours, chronic broncho-pneumonia germs die within 4 days, and typhoid-causing germs, which can also cause peritonitis, die within 5 days... these are much quicker times than can be claimed by modern antibiotics... what has happened to progress? Many eminent surgeons in hospitals all over the world declare that Honey makes a very effective and quick acting salve to apply with dressings after major surgery. It is also a very effective antibiotic for use with open wounds... wonderful Honey. Not only a fantastic healer of our outer bodies, Honey is also the best internal builder, strengthener, cleanser and healer in the world, it corrects

anything out of harmony or balance, Magic.
Let me list a few of the ways that honey can be used as a medicine and you will soon understand why it is that I plan one day to write Jennies Little Book of Honey Remedies!

Here goes:

Anaemia, abscesses, acidosis, alcoholism, angina-pectoris, arteriosclerosis, arthritis, asthma, bad-breath, biliousness, baldness, boils, bronchitis, bladder-stones, bedwetting, cataracts, catarrh, circulation, conjunctivitis, constipation, colitis, convulsions, cramps, coughs, dandruff, debility, diabetes, diarrhoea, dizziness, dropsy, dysentery, dyspepsia, eczema, emaciation, emotional upsets, energy-loss, fatigue, fevers, gallstones, gas, genito-urinary problems, goitre, gout, hair-loss, headaches, heart-weakness, headaches, haemorrhoids, high blood-pressure, hypoglycaemia, impotence, insomnia, indigestion, infections, influenza, irritability, jaundice, joint-pains, (including the so called growing pains of children), kidney-ailments, liver-ailments, low blood pressure, lumbago, lung-problems, malnutrition, menstrual cramps, mental-depression, muscle-weakness, nervousness, obesity, osteoporosis, pancreatitis, pleurisy, pneumonia, 'restless limbs', rheumatism, sterility, stomach-cramps, teeth and tongue problems, uric-acid build-up, voice hoarseness or loss, vomiting, worms and weight-problems can all be helped and the symptoms greatly alleviated by simply adding regular doses of Honey to the daily diet. The easiest and most pleasant way to take this most effective medicine, is simply to replace your normal tea or coffee drinks with honey and hot-water, WOW!

What a truly marvellous food-medicine this is .... Go and get some now! Take about a teaspoonful of honey in cup or mug of hot water the next time you need a 'cuppa' and not only will you be enjoying a good pick-me-up, you will also be treating your body to some of the tastiest and most efficacious medicine that it has ever had in its' life! By banishing tea, coffee and - sugar- from your store-cupboard, you will be helping yourself to health several times each day... Marvellous! And there's more! Just in case this list is not long enough, here is a list of ailments which can be healed by simply applying Honey externally as a salve, poultice or ointment....
Acne, alopecia, boils, burns, cold-sores, conjunctivitis, dermatitis, eczema,

face and body dryness, gum-problems, haemorrhoids, impetigo, insect-bites, lips cracking, nails splitting, pimples, psoriasis, spots, stings and wounds, What a life saver is a pot of Honey and all this for about a £1! There are yet more treasures in store in your Honey-jar, as there is no greater beautifier for the skin than Honey! Helen of Troy, Cleopatra, Madame de Pompadour and Elizabeth of Hungary are just a few of the famous beauties of history who used honey to ensure that their complexions stayed radiant and YOUNG.(Although Cleopatra bathed in asses milk, she used only Honey on her beautiful face and decreed that part of every marriage settlement should consist of a large Honey-gift to the bride!) Madame de Pompadour preferred her Honey to be whipped up in Champagne before using on her fabled complexion, and Elizabeth of Hungary mixed hers with Rosemary water, Helen used it neat!

Personally, I do not think that there are many cosmetics in the world, no matter what their prices, that can beat my favourite. Two teaspoonful of clear honey whipped up in 2 tablespoonful of Cornish cream and spread on the face quite liberally, will, if used regularly as a conditioning face-masque, soon have your skin looking like that of young girl and glowing with health. (Don't forget the golden rule with face packs 'THE FACE ENDS WHERE THE CAMISOLE BEGINS'.... this is one piece of Grandmamas advice which too many ladies seem never to have heard and their make-up line around the chin, prophecies a future 'wrinkly'!

The above mixture will keep in the refrigerator, but the substitution of 1 tablespoonful of olive oil and 1 tablespoonful of pure lemon juice, for the cream, will make a very effective beauty/massage cream, which will keep for as long as you wish, providing that it is in a screw-top jar or bottle. This mixture also makes a very effective scalp massage which clears dandruff, invigorates the scalp and promotes hair growth. Simply shake the mixture thoroughly then apply liberally to the scalp and massage in well, warm the head with a hairdrier or in front of the fire, cover with a towel and leave on for half an hour (now is the time to put your face pack on, sit with your feet in a bowl of hot water and drink a cup of herb or honey tea). Wash out with a herbal shampoo and your hair will be lustrous and sweet smelling, your skin and scalp clean and clear, your feet marvellous, nerves relaxed and you should be feeling totally rejuvenated! Magical Honey.

As Honey features so largely in my life, I have several ready prepared mixtures in my store-cupboard, which I make up at the weekends after shopping, the most widely used being a mixture of 3/4 honey to 1/4 cider vinegar, which I have bottled, all over the house, for use in just about every situation, for example:

In the kitchen I use it as my daily drink, with hot water added it is a great pep-up after shopping, housework, gardening, or any job which is energy-depleting..... In the 'fridge for use with cold water and ice, this is really delicious....In the bathroom as a conditioner after washing the hair, this is really good as it adjusts the PH balance of the hair-platelets, leaving it soft and silky, it is also often used in the bathwater as not only does it restore the acid mantle to the skin after bathing, but also acts as an aphrodisiac with its sweet sensuous aroma! It also proved very useful when my children were little as an instant 'cure' for all manner of bumps, bruises, cuts, stings, burns etc. and it had the added advantage of being 'lickable' if so desired! I think it is time to make up some for my daughter so that when little George-Brian starts perambulating, she will be well prepared for any emergency!

Another excellent mixture to keep in the store-cupboard is one of 1/4 Honey, 1/2 Olive Oil, and 1/4 Cider Vinegar. This mixture is a wonderful base which, with the addition of your favourite herbs, spices and condiments makes quick, tasty, healthy salad dressings, which not only enhance your culinary reputation, but also ease all manner of aches and pains into the bargain!

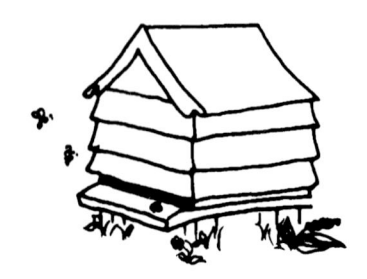

J is for Jam

Jam is reputed to be an instant source of nutrition at times when fresh fruit is unobtainable, but unfortunately that is not so of shop-bought jams due to an important and overlooked fact.

The most important asset to health which we obtain from fresh fruit is the action of its enzymes in converting the starches, sugars and proteins from that fruit into constituents of blood, bones, hormones, etc. a feat which it brings about without any change to itself and one which is really amazing, hence the 'apple a day.....' saying is true......
PROVIDED THE APPLE IS FRESH.BUT, as enzymes cannot function in extremes of heat or cold and work best between 32f and 104f and are destroyed by temperatures over 122f, and, as the boiling point of

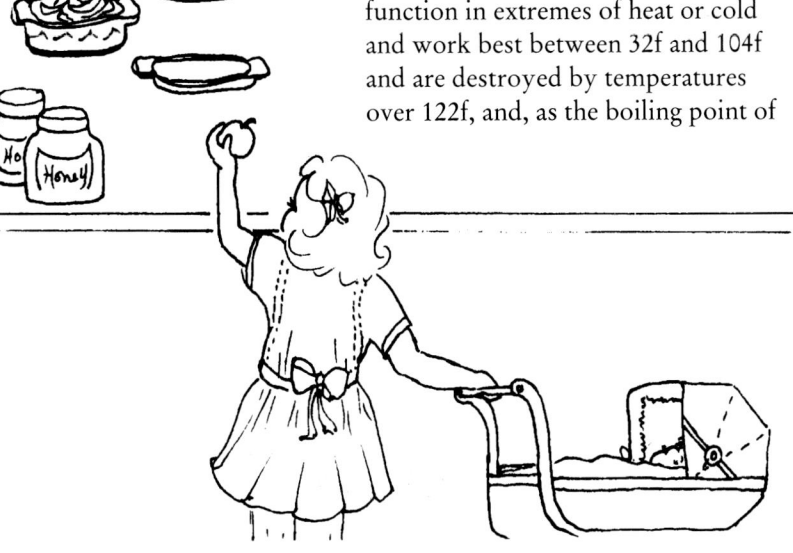

water is 212f you see that all vegetables and fruits lose their enzymes when they are boiled or stewed as in jam making. Nutritionists also know that vitamins cannot function without enzymes, so, without them also, what is left in jam? Not a lot! Only one more ingredient is featured in any quantity, and that is ... POISON... yes, you're learning, that tooth-rotting, hair-dropping, muscle-wasting, tissue-weakening, nerve-damaging yet most easily available of food poisons... SUGAR. Most of the other ingredients of jams, jellies, marmalades and pickles are either destroyed in the cooking or are chemicals, so these should not be in our homes. Oh dear... jam lovers must be despairing at this, but they can take heart for the answer lies in their own hands as it is quite easy to change to healthy alternatives... just read on...

One of the easiest ways I have found of making jam which still contains its' vitamins, minerals and enzymes is also one of the oldest ways known to Man (or should I say to Woman?) and can be made using any variety of fruit, in any amount, at any season, with none of the attendant hazards of traditional jam-making such as burned pans, scalds, wasps etc., I refer of course to the time-honoured tradition of compote-making. NO... I DID NOT SAY COMPOST MAKING! (I think that will be covered in Volume Sixty-seven at the rate I am going!)

To make a good compote, there are only a few things to remember and they apply equally to all fruits, marmalades and pickles:-

1) *Use only the best, fresh, ripe fruits, nuts or vegetables.*
2) *Use Honey as the only sweetener, don't poison with sugar.*
3) *Use equal weights of washed and seeded fruits and honey.*
4) *Mix well before putting into dish, cover with lid, NOT foil.*
5) *Use only glass or ovenproof china/stoneware for cooking.*
6) *Never have the oven heat above 100f. keep the enzymes alive.*
7) *Be patient, cook until reduced to half of the raw volume.*
8) *Keep out of reach of children if you want any for yourself!*

On the other hand, I always left them within easy reach of my children when they were little and most of my efforts were quickly snapped up by those mystery children who seem to live in the houses of all mothers with small children, and called' *I Dunno*', '*Nobody*' and '*Somebody else*'! Needless to say, although these never seen but always apparent children had the goodies, mine were the children who benefited from having the benefits of high-nutrition fruits all through the Winter months.

K is for Kelp

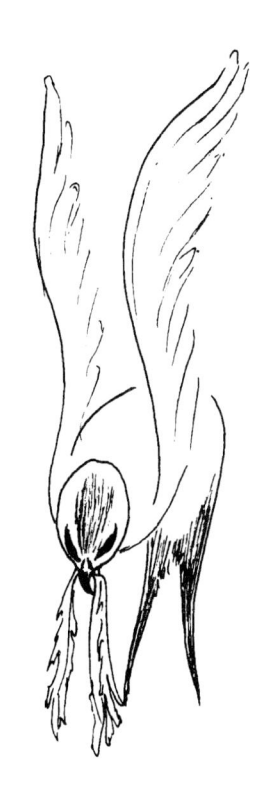

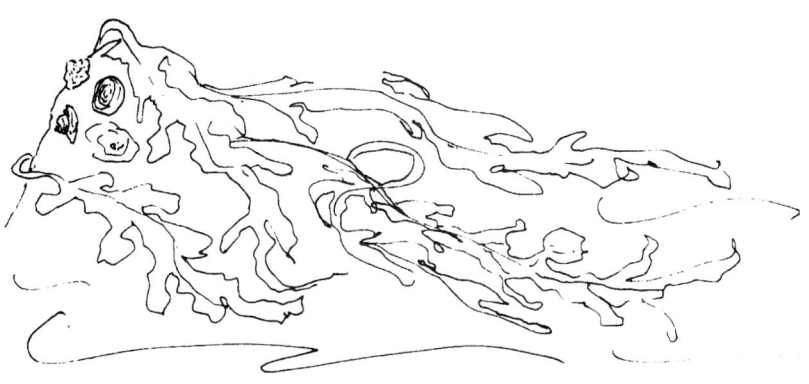

'Kelp'! you may exclaim, 'That's not a food"..... Well you would be wrong... Kelp is another of Mother Nature's miracle foods. Kelp contains not only Vitamins A, B, calcium, iron and phosphorus in goodly amounts, but also at least 60 trace elements which are essential for us to have in order to live a full and active life....Do you realise that it is quite possible for anyone to be full of energy and health right up to the minute they die? Not only is it possible, but in some cultures, where so-called civilisation' has not yet penetrated spreading its attendant legacy of ill-health and early death, it is the expected and a normal way of life! Yet here we are, an Island nation, not taking advantage of the wonderful health and life-giving Kelp, which grows around our shores, content to exist, instead of *really living*......well I for one am going to LIVE right up until the minute this body ceases to function and I leave this life! With Kelp in your store-cupboard you will be able to dish out this life, to all who eat at your table, and it is simplicity itself to use. Powdered kelp has a very pleasant taste and can be liberally sprinkled on any dish, which usually needs the addition of salt, soups, salads, meats and vegetables are all made tastier with the addition of this most valuable food. Kelp is the richest source of organic iodine and is especially helpful in cases of anaemia, brain-fatigue, diet-deficiency, diabetes, glandular problems including goitre, even impotency! What a wonderfully easy way to take your medicine...Go for Kelp, always use it at every meal and help yourself to good health.

One of the main benefits of Kelp is it's ability to help the body to assimilate all of the nutrients from other foods- something which we don't often manage due to the many toxins our bodies absorb during the course of our daily lives.

If you are one of the many people who eat well yet never seem to have enough energy, always feel tired at the end of the day yet never seem to sleep well, or suffer constantly from little niggling pains which are too unimportant to bother the doctor with yet cause enough discomfort to spoil your enjoyment of Life... take heart... and take Kelp.

Kelp is a highly nutritious and invaluable food medicine of which only a little is needed to do a lot of good, hence my advice to keep powdered Kelp on your table and use it daily as a condiment - you will soon feel much fitter if you do!

One special note for 'fatties' - and I have been one of you so no disrespect is intended - Kelp is one of the finest remedies for helping the body to rid itself of its excess fluid, and that includes the fluid surrounding the fat cells which create cellulite - what a wonderworker is Kelp! Get some today.

L is for Lemon

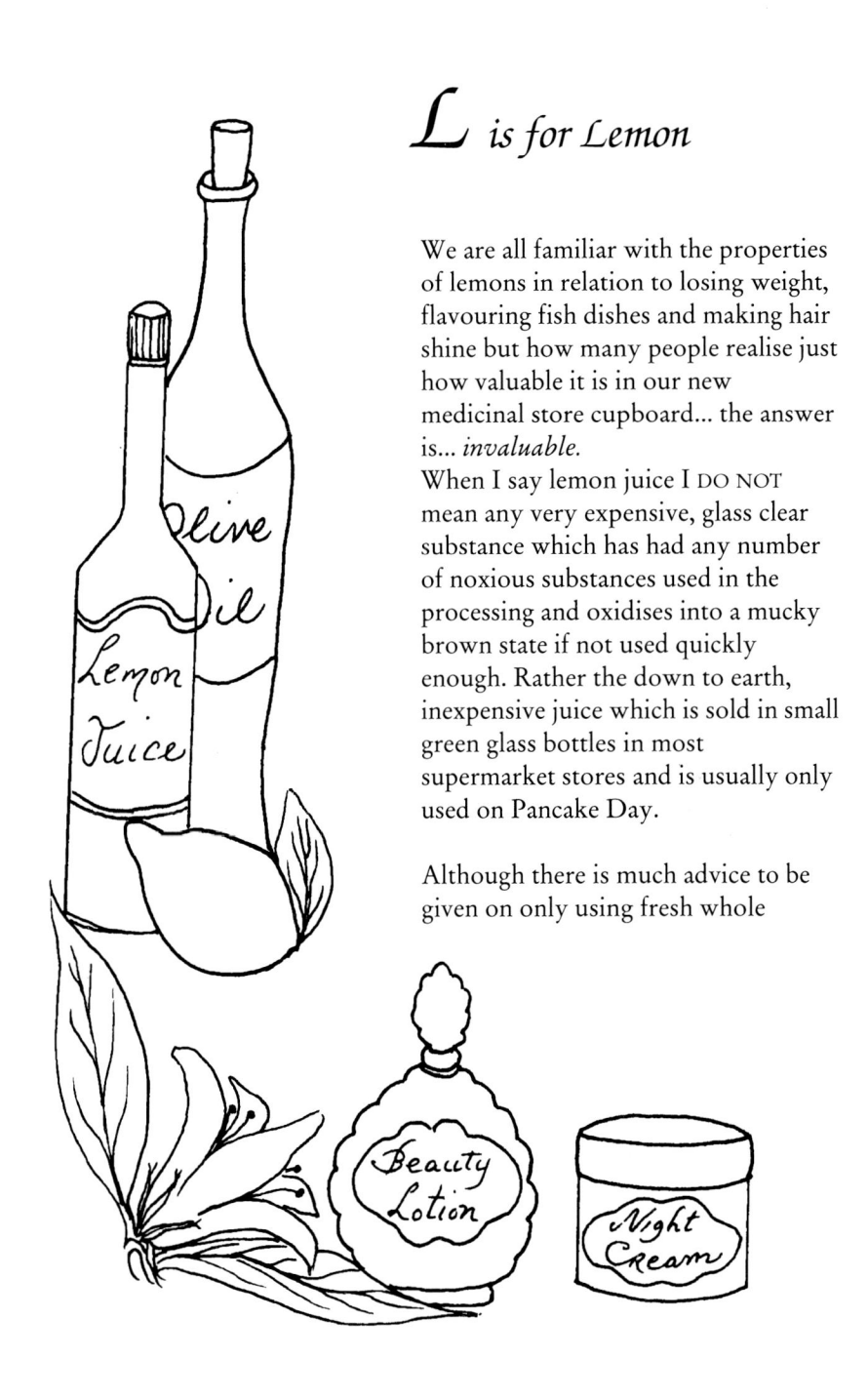

We are all familiar with the properties of lemons in relation to losing weight, flavouring fish dishes and making hair shine but how many people realise just how valuable it is in our new medicinal store cupboard... the answer is... *invaluable*.

When I say lemon juice I DO NOT mean any very expensive, glass clear substance which has had any number of noxious substances used in the processing and oxidises into a mucky brown state if not used quickly enough. Rather the down to earth, inexpensive juice which is sold in small green glass bottles in most supermarket stores and is usually only used on Pancake Day.

Although there is much advice to be given on only using fresh whole lemons, this is not an ideal world and most of us have to use whatever is available to us locally, regularly, at a price we can afford and as the bottled juice mentioned above, is a thousand times better than no lemon juice at all, then that is what I always have handy in my ever ready, health giving, medicinal store cupboard, and there are not many days when the little green bottle is not is use!

First and foremost must be its use in tea as a dissolvent for tannin and a taste-enhancer .....try it in place of milk the next time you have a 'cuppa' and you will be pleasantly surprised, also, if you do sometimes succumb to the odd cup of coffee now and then, a few drops of lemon juice added to a cup of black coffee, will take the edge off the bitterness of the cheaper blends. Also a little lemon juice in hot water makes a tasty drink, and, sweetened with honey makes an instant 'pick-me-up'.

Nature's Antiseptic, lemon juice will quickly destroy bacteria found in cuts, grazes and other small wounds giving anyone with small children a good reason to rush out and buy some. Did you know that lemon juice is also a very good remedy for insect bites and stings, blackhead, whiteheads, acne, eczema, erysipelas, (a skin disease formed by bacteria), sores, freckles, wrinkles, warts, corns and verruca? Well it is, and all you have to do is to apply it to the afflicted part and allow it to dry in, repeating the application at least three times daily until the problem has cleared..., what could be simpler?

Lemon juice also makes an excellent toothpaste if mixed with powdered sea-salt, which will even remove stubborn stains from smokers teeth, this 'toothpaste' (unlike some commercial sugar based products) is a good preventative of pyorrhea ,which brings early dentures, it also disinfects and strengthens the gums and freshens the breath at the same time, and all for a few pence!

Anyone who regularly suffers with sore throats, tonsillitis or quinsy would get much relief from gargling in a mixture of honey, lemon juice and hot water, to which a pinch of dried Sage has been added and allowed to steep for a few minutes.... This mixture can also be applied directly to the sore spots with a cotton swab and if applied several times daily after meals, will very speedily bring healing and comfort. I can vividly recall my Mother bringing me this tasty mixture when I was in bed with the 'flu, after which I promptly went to sleep and slept the clock around, waking fit, well, and full of energy!

Lemon juice, sniffed into the offending nostril is also an instant cure for nosebleed as I have proven on many an occasion with my family! Put onto warts, corns and verruca and allowed to dry, lemon juice is also quick and painless cure which is much less tear-inducing than conventional 'cut-out' methods! Sun-burned or wind-chapped skin is easily relieved and indeed improved, by the application of a mixture of equal parts of lemon juice, honey and olive oil, as a night cream.. when washing off, even after the first application, the skin appears to have gotten younger overnight.... lovely lemon juice! As lemon juice has antiseptic properties, I often recommend it to be used in the ratio of one teaspoonful, in a teacupful of warm water, as a vaginal or anal wash, in cases of vaginitis, pruritis, cystitis, itching haemorrhoids and similar complaints, it works speedily, bringing relief without tears or expense.

Of course, lemon juice really comes into its own in what my little friend Anna calls 'in our middles'. That region in the body which is governed by our orange/yellow vibrations and the part which decides the fate of the rest of our metabolism. From the lungs, through the stomach, spleen/pancreas, gall-bladder, kidneys, liver and intestines, lemon juice wending its way regularly, will assist the body in all of its functions, tending to prevent toxin build up, break down fatty acids, correct vitamin deficiencies, cleansing, strengthening and healing, particularly in cases of Arthritis, asthma, gall-bladder, liver and kidney problems, pneumonia, rheumatism, neuritis etc..!

Lemon, and in our case, lemon juice is absolutely invaluable, as it can be easily adapted in the kitchen either in food or drink.So if you suffer from any of the foregoing complaints try adding lemon juice to all of your recipes... it goes with just about anything excepting milk or cream and if you are a very good cook, you will even be able to blend lemon juice with them without curdling it ... I can't!

I do manage to make a Lemon-chiffon-custard which I have yet to fail on.(And if I can make it anyone can!) This is relished by anyone who tastes it and is extremely good for invalids, as it is both light, tasty and nutritious. Try some, I'm sure you'll love it:-

Soak 1 1/2 tablespoonfuls of gelatin in 1/2 cupful of cold water. Put 1pt (3/4ltr) of hot water, 4 tablespoonful of lemon juice and 4 tablespoonful of honey in a double boiler over hot water and bring back to the boil, then simmer until needed. Beat 4 egg yolks in a large bowl, then slowly pour the hot mixture into the eggs, stirring continuously until it thickens. Now add 1 teaspoonful of vanilla extract and the soaked gelatin and stir briskly for about 2 minutes. When this cools and begins to set, beat together with an egg yolk until smooth and thick, pour into individual dishes and leave to set in the refrigerator for several hours. Served with a swirl of whipped cream with a garnish of finely grated lemon-peel and a drizzle of honey. This dish is surely the Ambrosia of the Gods.... and what a super way to help yourself to health! Make sure that YOU have lemon juice.

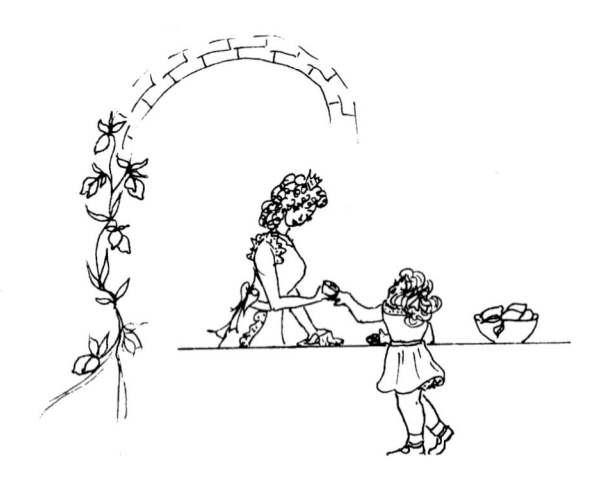

$\mathcal{L}$ is for Lentils

A lot of rude jokes are made about lentils, also a lot of rubbish is written about the absolute necessity of including them in the diet of anyone who is vegetarian.... I will try to 'strike the happy medium' by only giving you the advice I would use myself... as I have done all through this little book and the others in the series.

Lentils are indeed a very nourishing food, containing Vitamins A, B-Complex, C, Calcium, Iron and Phosphorus. They are a good body building food and as such are highly recommended in cases of low blood pressure, anaemia, colitis and anorexia, and other debilitating illnesses where strength is needed in order to fight fatigue. For example, Debility, Emaciation, Muscle weakness, M.E.,

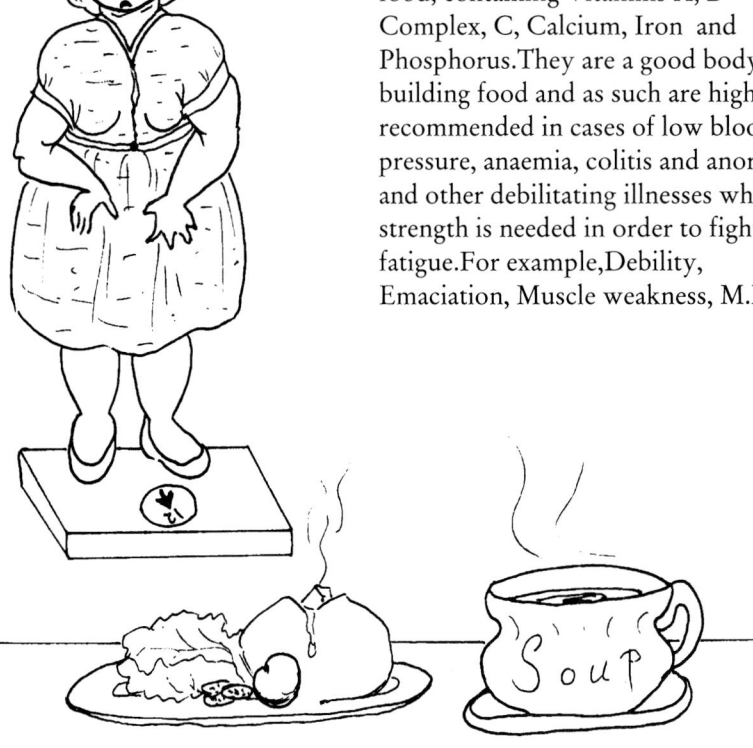

Lethargy, M.N.D., Internal Ulcerative conditions, etc. As lentil soup is so easily made simply by boiling the lentils for a few hours together with your favourite vegetables and herbs, even the poorest cook should keep lentils in their store cupboard as a standby in case of illness (or indeed just as a tasty health food to keep you in peak condition!) Go Spanish with your lentils by cooking up 1 cup of Lentils to 1 1/4 pts (1ltr) water until they are tender, then adding 2 cups of chopped tomatoes, 1 finely chopped Spanish onion, 1 chopped green pepper, 1 teaspoonful of Cornflour, 1 large pinch each of sea salt, ground celery and marjoram and simmering until tender and the tastes have 'melded' ..... this should be about an hour by which time your taste buds should be watering... its delicious.

Another tasty way of having lentils is to take 1 cup of lentils which have been soaked overnight and add 1 small chopped onion, 1 teaspoonful of dried parsley, 1 cup of chopped celery, 1 large chopped potato, 1 large chopped carrot, 1 sliced lemon, a few cloves and a pinch of black pepper .Cook in 1 1/4 pts (1ltr) of water until the potatoes are tender then put through the liquidiser and serve topped with a swirl of cream, a knob of butter or a thin slice of lemon sprinkled with parsley. If it is a little thick, a little warm milk can be added to make an unusual, piquant and very nourishing meal, one of my special favourites. Don't forget though... Lentils are a body builder, so if you are trying to lose weight, have this IN PLACE of a meal! Too many people are overweight because they under estimate the nourishment in a bowl of soup and eat a meal as well... don't let this happen to you, Lentils are a body building medicine.

While on the subject of lentils, I feel that it should be mentioned that Split peas, dried marrowfat peas, chick-peas, butter, lima and other species of dried beans, all contain similar properties and help to heal and rebuild the body and as such should be included in the diet of anyone suffering from any debilitating illness as often as possible,... BUT... one word of warning... when soaking *red kidney beans* overnight, ALWAYS strain the soaking water away and rinse in cold water *before* boiling in fresh water, and ALWAYS boil fast, for at least 20 minutes, before lowering the heat to simmer. This ensures that no toxicity remains and you help yourself to helpings of health.

M is for Molasses

Molasses is the only thing of any nutritional value to come from the sugar cane.. The starchy mess which is left after the extraction, should be labelled with the skull and crossbones, before being disposed of but unfortunately, it is instead treated with several lethal chemicals, bleached, dried and separated into grains, then bagged and sold as ... SUGAR!

Molasses contains many vitamins, minerals and trace elements and is an absolutely indispensable medicine food for anyone suffering from constipation, diverticulitis, irritable bowel, and all similar complaints which stem from 'clogged workings'.

If any of us needed speedy relief from constipation as young children, we

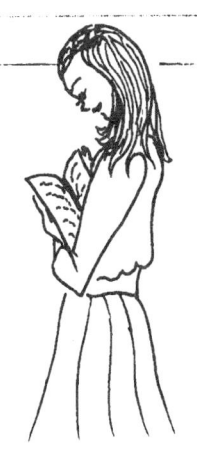

were simply given a glass of hot milk with a teaspoonful of molasses to stir into it in place of our evening meal... the next morning the queue for the loo told Grandmama, that no more medicine would be needed in the near future! I have also found that if young children are fed with molasses fairly regularly they do not even get constipated.... simplicity itself. To make this helps anyone with slow digestion. Into a large mixing bowl put:-
1lb. (500gms) wholemeal flour, 1 lb, (450gms) medium oatmeal, 2 tsps. baking powder, a pinch of sea salt and mix well. In a small saucepan warm together 6ozs vegetable lard, 6ozs honey, 6ozs molasses, add to the dried mixture and beat well for one minute, adding enough milk to make into a stiff batter. Pour into a grease papered tin and bake for about an hour in a moderate oven. When cool... HIDE!

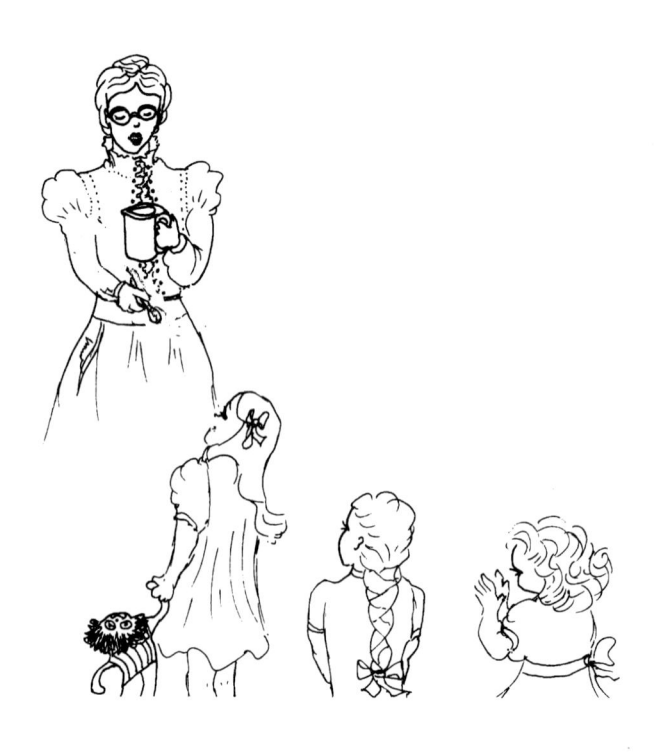

$\mathcal{N}$ is for Nuts

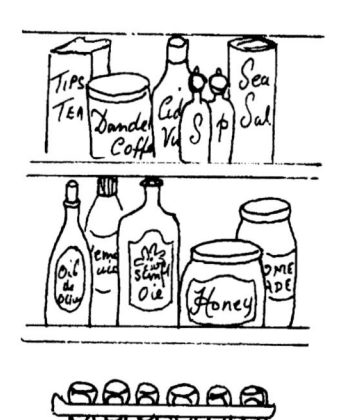

There are many kinds of nuts, all of which contain many mineral and vitamin nutrients and are rich in natural carbohydrates making them a valuable addition to the medicinal store-cupboard but, there are one or two important things to remember about nuts... the edible kind, not the people like me kind!

While most nuts have an alkaline reaction on the system, peanuts, hazelnuts or filberts and walnuts, are acid forming, so anyone who is careful about combining their foods correctly, which is an important health move, should watch their nuts! On the whole, nuts are excellent food medicines for anyone suffering from faulty metabolism, muscle and body weakness and in fact, any wasting, tiring, or deteriorating sickness. What

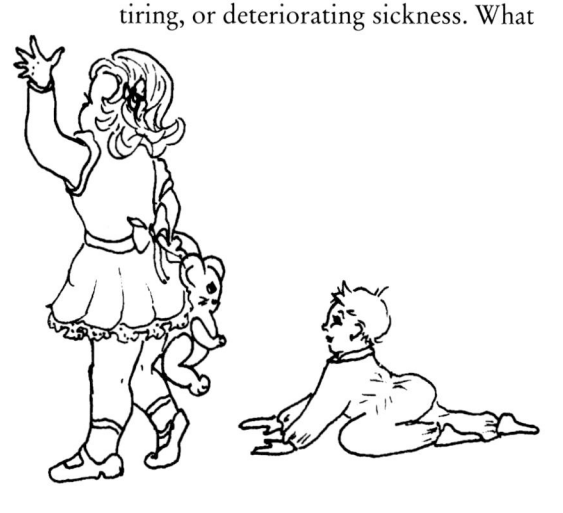

53

wonderful foods to have in our store cupboards, yet how seldom most people make use of them. Well, that's over now that you know how good for you nuts can be isn't it?.. 'Yes Jennie'!

Too often we forget how versatile the nut can be. Try putting a cupful of nuts into your grinder and adding this nut-flour to any cooking you may do for an elderly or infirm person, their cooking will then be health foods.. try also adding this fine nut-flour to breakfast cereals, pies, cakes and puddings, etc. Also 1 dessertspoonful, mixed to paste with a little milk, then topped up with hot milk, makes a deliciously different and strength giving drink for an invalid too poorly to eat a meal. If this drink is sweetened with honey and sprinkled with nutmeg it makes a nutritious, soothing, sleep promoting bed time drink.

Rough ground nuts are nicer with salads, cookies and ice cream and, as most children love nuts, are a quick and tasty energy booster and a boon to the nutrition conscious, busy mother. As we use such a lot of Honey in this house, there are always plenty of screw-topped jars around, so I keep my nuts in these jars after shelling and grinding them fresh for when I need them. Mothers with small children can be sure that their little ones will appreciate their thoughtfulness in grinding a variety of nuts at the same time and storing them on a low shelf, in the refrigerator until needed in air-tight jars. I used to keep my jars well within reach of little people, knowing full well that they were helping themselves to instant energy any time they felt the need... but.. don't forget the golden rule with children.... NEVER SAY 'EAT BECAUSE IT IS GOOD FOR YOU', that is the one thing that will put paid to all your good intentions regarding healthy eating.... children HATE anything labelled 'good, sensible' etc. they love 'quickies, treats, or forbidden' foods, so be crafty and they'll be fit!

Another wonderfully easy to prepare meal and one packed full of goodness, is made by simply chopping either a grapefruit, orange or tangerine and adding to a small handful of figs or dates, arranging on a bed of lettuce leaves, watercress or any other shredded greens and decorating with slices of red, green or yellow peppers add a sprinkling of chopped, sliced or whole nuts... This salad can be made to look very attractive, by the careful arrangement and colour blending of the ingredients and is appreciated, especially by 'liverish' people and anorexics.

Of course, no chapter on nuts would be complete without a page on that most versatile of health foods, the 'meat' of many vegetarians and vegans and the boon to busy mothers...

Peanuts! Having as they do, a very high protein and calorie content, and having a high fat content also, peanuts are one of the most nourishing and body building foods available and have the added advantage of being easy to eat and, relatively inexpensive. (A feature which is becoming more and more important in these days of high inflation and low incomes, problems which face us all). In order to get the best benefit from your peanuts, buy them fresh. (Do make sure that you do not get the red-skinned variety, as these need peeling before eating, as the red skins contain chemicals which are harmful, particularly for asthmatics, and indeed, anyone suffering with respiratory troubles, also young children who can so easily choke when eating.)

Peanuts contain many of the B-Complex vitamins, together with Calcium, iron, phosphorus, potassium and Vitamin E and are also rich in trace elements and have the added benefits that they are universally accepted by young and old alike as a 'taster' rather that a health food, so are more likely to be eaten often. Peanut butter is easily made by grinding the nuts with a little sea salt then mixing to a paste with the addition of a very little peanut, sunflower, or any other vegetable oil.... I have a friend who mixes hers with sunflower margarine and it has a lovely light texture, I personally prefer the rough ground nuts mixed with a little olive oil and a smidgen of yeast extract or powdered kelp and my children used to say it was yummylicious!

O is for Oil

There are many types of oil available in shops and supermarkets and all of them are better for use in cooking, than animal fats, but some oils are much more beneficial than other. It is these medicinal oils, which we should have in our store cupboards, particularly Sunflowerseed, Grapeseed and Olive oils.

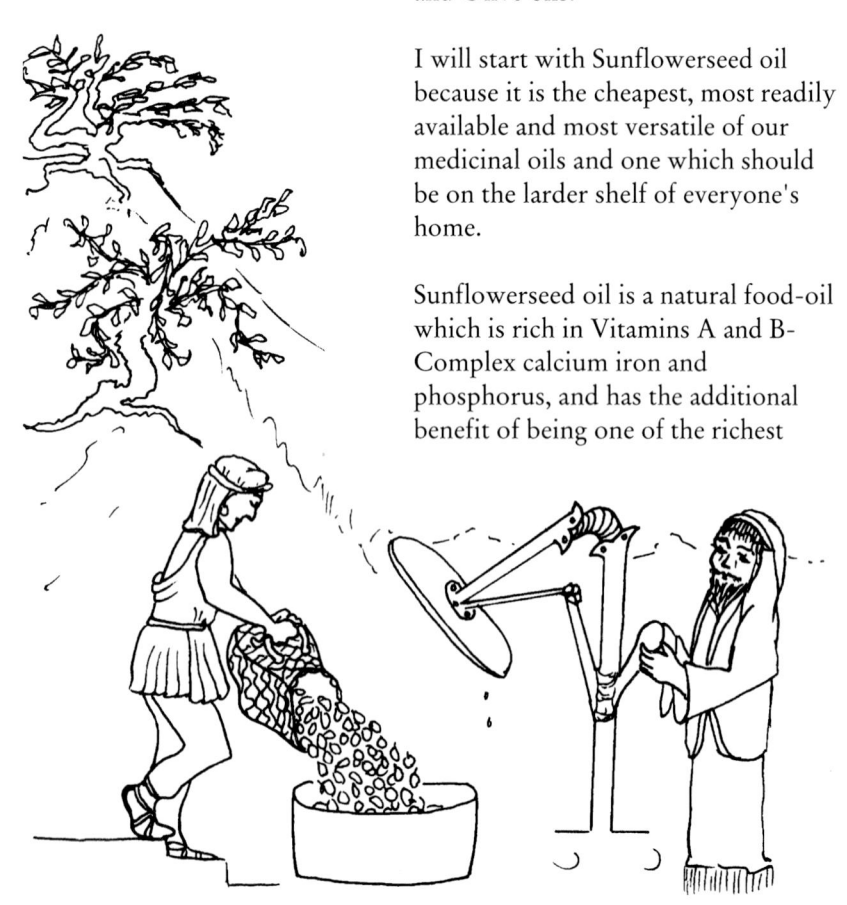

I will start with Sunflowerseed oil because it is the cheapest, most readily available and most versatile of our medicinal oils and one which should be on the larder shelf of everyone's home.

Sunflowerseed oil is a natural food-oil which is rich in Vitamins A and B-Complex calcium iron and phosphorus, and has the additional benefit of being one of the richest sources of Vitamin E, the youth vitamin. HOWEVER, as vitamin E is partly destroyed by refining and by heating for any length of time, the oil must be COLD-PRESSED in order for us to obtain the full benefit. If your grocer does not stock cold-pressed oil, either ask him to get some in for you or shop around until you find some. The benefit to your health will make it well worth the effort, as cold-pressed sunflowerseed oil nourishes the whole body, feeding and repairing the body cells, tissues and organs, strengthening eyesight, nails and tooth enamel, lubricating the joints, moisturising and beautifying the skin, and all we have to do to obtain such benefits, is to include this versatile oil for frying, roasting, baking, and salad-dressing etc. in the store-cupboard Marvellous! What an easy way to help ourselves to better health isn't it?

Grapeseed oil is a lovely light, slightly nutty oil which contains slightly less vitamin E than other oils, but more than makes up for that lack, by its' richness in other vitamins, minerals and particularly traces of organic acids, which are so very valuable to anyone suffering from Arthritis, constipation, gout, kidney and liver disorders, psoriasis, rheumatism and indeed, any disorder caused by faulty elimination of toxins.

Grapeseed oil can be used in the same way as any other oil in the kitchen, but it also has the benefit that because it is so light, it can be used as the base for many potions and lotions and applied externally for the relief of aches and pains. Try putting a few sprigs of crushed Rosemary into a bottle of grapeseed oil and keeping in a warm, handy place to use as an embrocation to relieve chesty coughs, arthritic joints, gouty limbs, menstrual cramps, windy stomachs and in fact anywhere that the pain is caused by a hang-up in the circulation. Relief is not long in coming, and what other medicine has the added advantage that it tastes delicious when poured over lamb and roasted, used to flavour soups or added to salad dressing?

As grapeseed oil also contains anti-depressant and relaxant properties, I find it very useful to have a small bottle handy, to which I have added, a large pinch of ground Mace or Nutmeg. Both of which are marvellous for soothing the nervous system. So a little of this oil, rubbed into the soles of the feet or the palms of the hands quickly lifts the spirits and soothes the troubled mind... this is also a good remedy for insomnia.

Olive oil must surely be everyone's favourite. As its' rich nutty flavour goes so well with a variety of foods and indeed tastes good enough to take by itself... I love Olive oil and do so wish, that everyone could be made aware of its' benefits, so that everyone makes sure that it is in their store cupboard. First and foremost let me stress again,that the very best bodies, deserve only the very best oil and that must surely be Pure *Cold-Pressed Extra-Virgin Olive Oil*... my Husband says that any thing with a name like that, must be a thing to treasure in this day and age!.. he jokes, but I agree with him, as this health food is indeed a treasure in any age and for people of any age. Olive oil stimulates the contractions of the gall-bladder, so that anyone suffering from any gall-bladder problems can take heart, and take olive oil for their cooking instead of simply resigning themselves to a fry-free life! This is a particular boon to men who hate the idea of living on bland food yet suffer with gall-bladder, liver, pancreas or digestive problems. Olive oil lubricates the joints when regularly taken internally, this is also marvellous for anyone suffering from Arthritis, fibrositis, frozen joints, gout, rheumatism etc. Volume 1 in this series contains a great many remedies which can be made using Olive oil as a base, but as this book is primarily a *food remedy* book, may I suggest you try one of my favourite and most simple food remedies for any of the foregoing problems:

Take one OVEN BAKED jacket potato, (microwaves destroy vitamins), cut open, mash the inside with a fork and dress with Olive oil, sea salt and black pepper and eat every bit.Very simple and   Food for the Gods!

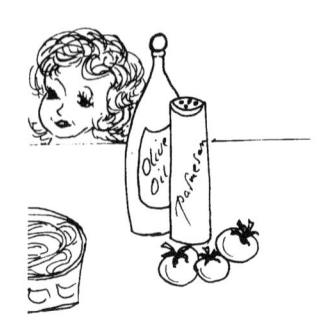

$\mathcal{P}$ is for Pasta

Pasta surprisingly is very rich in vitamins and minerals and, as made with pure durum wheat, has wheat's good properties and so can be a very useful addition to the diet, especially where there are teenagers who have an aversion to 'proper' food and who welcome anything with a continental flavour... if you can't beat them join them, as the saying goes, but in the process make sure that they are in reality joining you... Just make sure that the pasta is of the finest quality, the ingredients to complement it are fresh, the herbs and spices used to flavour the dishes are carefully selected and you will be amazed at how much good you can do by simply cooking up a 'with-it' meal!

Pasta covers a wide variety, Spaghetti, macaroni, vermicelli, tagliatelle, lasagne, etc., and comes in many shapes and sizes, hoops, twists, shells, strands etc., yet all pastas are good health-giving ingredients and should be used regularly in our health and fitness programme. I think that it is marvellous to be able to throw any mixed vegetables into a pan to stir-fry, meanwhile boiling up the pasta, strain then mix together, and serve up a dish which is usually enjoyed by all and sundry!

Everyone from tots to teens, students to senior citizens, and groupies to grannies can benefit from having the addition of regular tasty pasta meals to their diets, and, one of the most attractive things about it to my mind, is the fact that, in an emergency, with the addition of a few cans or some eggs and cheese, a nutritious and tasty meal can be made in half an hour which will satisfy even the most critical gastronome... with small or teenaged children, no home is complete without Pasta!

One of my children's favourite pasta recipes is cooked in no time, uses up any vegetables to hand and is always received and enjoyed by all who taste it! Here is my 'fail safe' recipe:-

Into a large pan of boiling salted water, put 2-3ozs of pasta per person and cook as directed on the packet. While cooking, finely chop any vegetables which you have to hand - carrots, courgettes, tomatoes, peppers, mushrooms, onions, leeks, garlic, celery, broccoli etc. and fry in a little olive oil for about three minutes. Add enough vegetable stock to create a tasty gravy; strain the pasta and pour the mixture over for a very tasty quick meal which disappears in no time and is very nutritious.

Any type of flavouring may be used to vary this dish.

My son has on occasion made his 'special' by frying a mixture of fruits and using fruit juice as gravy, thus producing a marvellous and warming dessert in winter which, as a finishing touch, was drizzled over with honey - it sounds odd but tastes delicious!

So don't be afraid to experiment with your pasta!

$\mathcal{P}$ is for Pepper

Pepper is in most store cupboards and again is usually one of the most under rated food medicines, as we are constantly being advised *not* to use seasonings on our food. However, if we use pure black peppercorns and grind them at the table when we need them, we will be helping ourselves to health every time we indulge in this tasty food medicine.

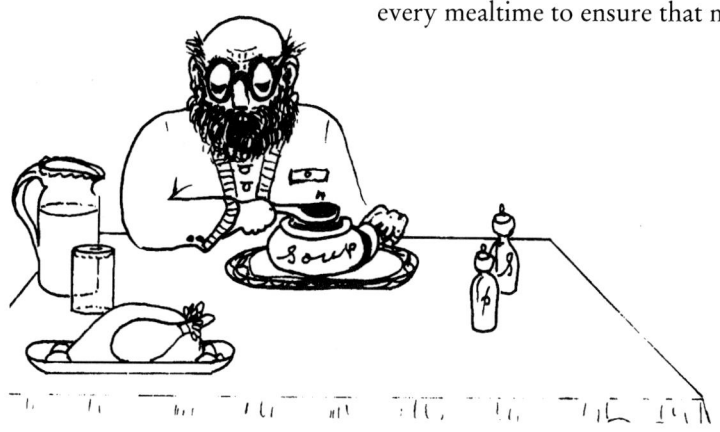

Black peppercorns are readily available today and are fairly inexpensive, not as they were in the time of Atilla the Hun who demanded 3,000 lbs of peppercorns in ransom for the city of Rome.... they must have been worth their weight in gold then and I often used to wonder as a child, whatever did he do with them? I do nothing much with mine, excepting use them at every mealtime to ensure that my tissues are stimulated into action, thus helping to guard against the so-common women's' complaints such as prolapse of the bladder, rectum or womb.

During my coffee drinking period, I also developed high blood pressure, which needed to be controlled for many years with high risk medication and its' attendant side effects. But due to a few well-chosen herbs and peppercorns' regulating action, I now keep it at a manageable level without having to resort to drugs. This truly is a remarkable medicine food, not only for its regulating effect on the blood but also for the way that it helps the body to eliminate toxic waste more effectively, thus bringing ease from the discomforts which attend elimination hang-ups. A wonderful hot remedy to cool the system is Pepper!

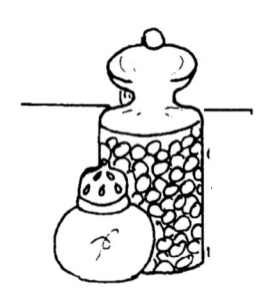

$\mathcal{R}$ is for Rice

Rice is nice, brown rice is nicer, wild brown rice is the best. In our new health enhancing store cupboard we should always keep some of the best rice as a good standby for emergencies as it contains appreciable amounts of the B-Complex vitamins plus vitamin K, calcium, iron, phosphorus and potassium, which, added to the fact that it is one of the most easily digested starches which provides all of the necessary carbohydrate requirements for good health, makes it an almost miraculous food medicine, and with its added benefit of versatility, one which we should not only keep handy but also use regularly!

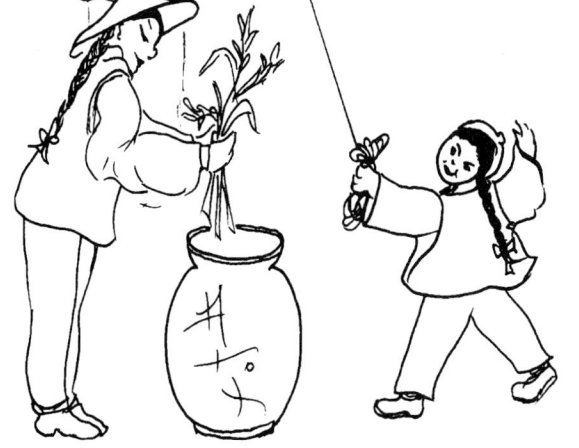

Another of the body-building foods, rice is the staple diet of the majority of Asiatic countries, where, were we to believe in its ancient reputed value as an aphrodisiac and fertility food, we would say that living proof of its efficacy is everywhere!

While I was living in Sri Lanka and working in the hospital there, it amazed me at first to see visitors give the patients parcels wrapped up in banana leaves which, when they were opened proved to contain cooked rice with various flavourings. However, once I had started to go out and about and visit the eating places which were frequented by the Singhalese and had sampled the indigenous meals, most of which has this wild rice as their base, I no longer wondered at the eagerness with which these oriental 'meals on wheels' were greeted...... I no longer ate in the tourist hotels either, but made my 'local' a cafe where the main rice-based meals were served on banana leaves!

Surprisingly, I did not put on any weight with my high energy carbohydrate fare and felt full of energy and able to cope with any problems which came my way in the course of my working day. Have you ever wondered why it is the Asiatics and Orientals seem to take everything in their stride and hardly ever get uptight about anything? Maybe the anti-stress factors of their diet have something to do with it, not least being the relaxant properties of vitamin K coupled with very low meat consumption. Western nations suffer terribly from stress and their diets contain the highest concentration of meats and sugars anywhere in the world.... need I say more?

Our grandmothers knew what they were doing when they served up rice puddings and such like. The old-fashioned rice pudding which we all remember from our childhood and which has been superseded by a variety of empty 'instant' concoctions mainly comprising sugar and chemicals, is still one of the easiest and tastiest ways of getting good nutrition into a sick person who cannot take a full meal, and, as mentioned in Volume One of this series, when topped with a sprinkling of nutmeg to soothe the nerves, becomes a champion remedy for digestive problems, including stomach and intestinal ulcers, flatulence, colic and cramps, plus that scourge of the sickroom, diarrhoea.

Insomniacs will also have cause to call down blessings on your head if you make them a little dish of rice pudding with Nutmeg or Mace sprinkled on the top for supper as this will ensure that they get a good nights' sleep, and, as the only time that cells can repair themselves is during sleep, this spells Health.

Rice is very versatile and there are many ways in which it can be used for cooking and, as I would not insult you by telling you how to cook a rice pudding, let me instead share with you some of the ways in which I used to cook it for my children thus ensuring them strong healthy bones, muscles, teeth and nails, with healthy, shining eyes and beautiful gleaming hair. Rice-pies were a firm favourite and much more in demand than traditional pies with a pastry case and were very simply made by lining a baking dish with hot boiled rice, then filling with a mixture of:-

A) Onions, tomatoes, red beans, peppers and Oregano;
B) Cauliflower, leeks, cheese, chives and Celerysalt;
C) Mushrooms, sweetcorn, peas, carrots and Coriander;
D) Boiled eggs, spinach, parsnip, swede and Cinnamon;
E) Courgettes, peppers, apples, coconut and Curry;
F) Baked mixed beans, leeks, tomatoes and Chillies;
(This last is a great favourite with youngsters and can be made with any types of canned beans or even pastas in an emergency!) Cover with more rice and cook in a moderate oven for 30 minutes. As you can see, there are many combinations and I suggest that you experiment with the foods which you think that your family would like... as I am vegetarian there is no meat recipe but you could add whichever meat or fish you like to each dish, just adjusting the cooking times as necessary... and then watch your efforts disappear at the meal table...as for desserts,the possibilities are endless, do try some rice-pies for yourself and help yourself to health using the Healers in YOUR home.

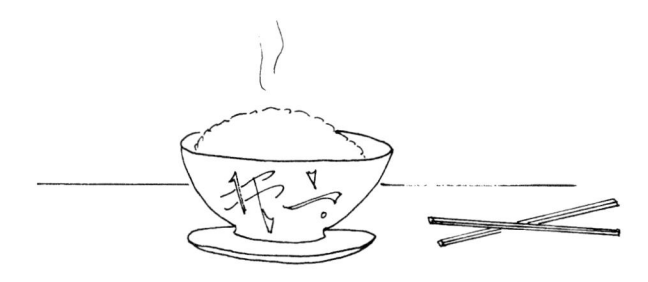

S is for Salt

Sea Salt is good for you, Rock salt is bad...
So if you are one of the millions of people who are suffering from a bland food diet because you were unaware that there was a difference, take heart, and take *sea salt*.

Sea salt helps your body fluids to move regularly through the system in a similar manner to the ebb and flow of the sea. Rock salt on the contrary, keeps fluids static and still in between the tissues similar to its' appearance in its' natural habitat.

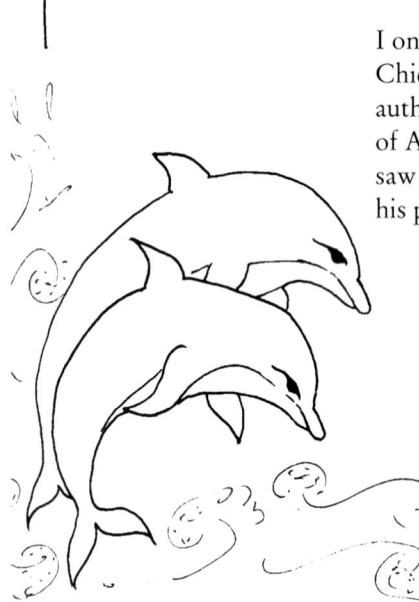

I once worked with Dr. O Janes of Chicago, (one of the worlds' leading authorities on the prevention and cure of Arthritis by natural methods) and saw some quite remarkable results of his policy of ensuring that all arthritic patients, took large daily doses of Sea salt and also added it to their bathwater.

If you or anyone you know suffers from Arthritis, fibrositis, gout, rheumatism or associated complaints, try adding sea salt to your daily diet. Also adding a handful of sea salt to the bathwater each time you have a bath and gently exercising the affected limbs under the water, I'm sure will make you feel better.

Iodised sea salt is even better for the system, as Iodine is one of the most important natural minerals for healthy survival, and one that is only available from the sea. and, As we as a nation, do not eat nearly enough seafood, iodised sea salt has a good supply and will be most beneficial for anyone suffering from Thyroid deficiency, slow metabolism, fatigue, obesity etc.

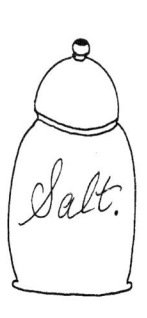

S is for Sardines

Sardines are one of the few tinned foods I always keep handy in my store cupboard. They are one of the best, vitamin and mineral foods available, making a tasty snack in seconds and ensuring that the calcium and phosphorus reservoirs of the body, do not get depleted, so guarding against the onset of osteoporosis. The womenfolk in our family all have a tendency to this 'shrinking syndrome' (Father always said that Aunt Edie had to be buried in a tea-chest because she had shrunk so much!) and, as I am only 5ft tall if I stand on a sixpence I can't afford to shrink as I grow older, so I have a can of sardines once a week. This is no hardship to me, as they are one of my favourite foods, but if you do not like them, yet feel that you may be prone to osteoporosis, you could try mixing them with cider vinegar and rolling them in lettuce leaves; popping them in soups or stews where the taste disappears; mixing into any herby or spicy dish or of course having them the Italian way as follows:-

Saute 3 or 4 cloves of Garlic in a tablespoonful of olive oil until golden, then add a can of tomato puree or chopped plum tomatoes, a can of sardines, a pinch of basil, a little sea salt and ground black pepper and simmer for 15-20 minutes. Cook about 4-6ozs spaghetti twists or similar pasta for about 15 minutes or as directed on the packet, then drain, add a little butter and serve topped with the sauce and chopped parsley... Mmm I do like taking food medicine, it sure beats pills and potions and hopefully this one will stop me from shrinking away!

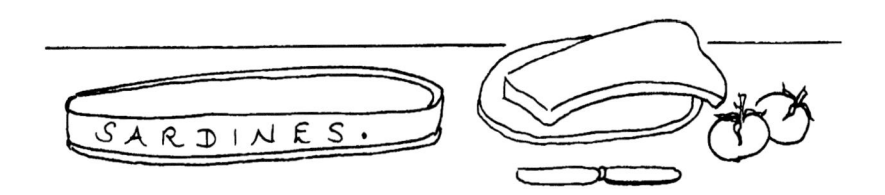

S is for Sugar

If ever there was a non-food which should carry a Government health warning and perhaps have the skull and crossbones as its' emblem, that product should surely be....SUGAR... Non-beneficial to the body, nerve-destroying, life-shortening, habit-forming, bone-decaying, addictive SUGAR. probably as addictive in its' effect, as many hard core drugs, and most of us actively encourage our children into addicts by the time they are seven years of age!

'Not me' you may say. But unless you can say to yourself with your hand on your heart, that you *do not* have SUGAR in your store cupboard, *do not* buy any product labelled 'natural preservative', *have never* given sweets, chocolates or toffee's as a treat, and neither smoke, or drink carbonated beverages... then the chances are, that you not only actively encourage all in your household to be 'sugar takers', but are in fact yourself a SUGARHOLIC!

If you think I exaggerate the addictive properties of SUGAR then just throw away any SUGAR or foods containing SUGAR and try to manage to exist, for a whole week, on foods and drinks with absolutely no added sugar, and that includes *cigarettes!*

Absentmindedness, bad breath, colds, diarrhoea, emphysema, fury, griping, hot and cold flushes, hallucinations, itching, irritability, joint pains, kidney pains, lips chapping, muscle cramps, nervousness etc. etc. are just some of the symptoms of SUGAR-WITHDRAWAL which can be expected.... sounds just like any other drug-addict going 'cold turkey' doesn't it? SUGAR CAN KILL. Get rid of this 'POISON' from your store cupboard for all time.

If you have small children who have a 'sweet tooth', gradually introduce Honey into their diets in place of sugar. This way you will be feeding them Good Health.

Try making Honey treats to replace the sugar - filled snacks which children are so fond of, they are easy to make, delicious to eat and relatively inexpensive.

Mix any grated nuts, dried fruits and grains with enough honey to make a fairly stiff mixture, form into balls and put on a greased baking tray and cook in a moderate oven for about 20 minutes. Allow to get completely cold before taking off the tray - Store in an airtight tin and use as a treat instead of 'sugar snacks.

$\mathcal{T}$ is for Tea

Tea... picked by nimble fingers in the brilliant sunshine on the mountain slopes of far-flung and exotic countries, then carried across the oceans of the world for our sheer enjoyment... What pictures that conjures up in the imagination and how true they used to be in the days when speed had not become so important. When I was in India and Ceylon, I visited the tea plantations and followed the production of tea from the plantation to the pot and found out some very pertinent facts about our national tipple, some of which are very important to anyone who is trying to help themselves to health via their store cupboard.

Come with me to the hillside of Sri Lanka and see the pickers with their colourful saris delicately picking the

tea leaves from the rows of glistening plants.
First the tips, the youngest, most delicate leaves are picked and placed into pouches on the front of the pickers saris, then the next leaves down the stem are picked and put with a graceful over-arm movement into baskets which hang from the pickers heads and rest on their backs, these two pickings are the 'pick of the crop' if you'll excuse the pun, and when dried, are used to make some of the finest teas in the world. Then the lower, older, drier leaves are picked and put into large sack-like receptacles hanging from the pickers waists, leaving trails of denuded plants in the wake of the pickers as they wend their way down the rows and towards the drying racks where the sun-dried leaves soon become their familiar tea-colour.

In the drying sheds the teas are carefully placed in their separate lots, graded, inspected, sieved, flavoured and in some
instances coloured, before being packed into chests for shipping. BUT despite tea vendors protests to the contrary, no grain of tea is wasted... every gramme counts... and any leaves, chippings or dust which may have fallen on to the floor, is very carefully swept up and put into the chests which contain the large leaves from the last picking. Believe me...I was there! Loose leaf tea tips makes a refreshing cuppa and does us good. These 'tips' contain all the relaxant or stimulant properties of the tea plant according to which variety is harvested. These are usually reserved for the very best quality teas. Even the second pick or full-leaf tea can still taste good and do you good, this is usually used for those branded teas which are regularly advertised on the television and carry the name of the companies which own the factories and shipping depots in the countries where the plantations are; BUT and here we come to the crunch... the last picking with its older, tougher, tannin-filled leaves with the stems, twigs (and sometimes even floor-sweepings) are ground up, coloured, treated, and used for putting into tea-bags, especially the cheaper and 'own brands'! (incidentally, in order to produce the paper to make tea-bags, trees are rotted quickly in special lagoons, and treated with chemicals to break down their fibre in half of the normal time, so is it any wonder that we now die in half the time we used to?) If you drink tea bag tea voluntarily after reading this, you do not deserve to be called a tea-drinker... rather a toxin- taker!

Personally I much prefer a good old-fashioned 'cuppa' made in the pot and left to stand until it is a rich golden-brown with a twist of lemon or a smidgen of honey to enrich the taste. Rather than that dreadful bag, dunked in the cup and leaching that horrible orange stain into the water... and as for milk in tea... Well, what can I say except that I like tea to taste of tea not like baby food! Seriously though milk reacts badly with tannin and creates an acid imbalance in the stomach so if you suffer from recurring bouts of tummy-trouble, try taking your tea without milk and see what relief you get.

There are many medicinal teas available in the supermarkets today which should be in your larder in case of emergencies, try Bergamot for stress, tension or depression; Earl Grey with lemon and honey for shortness of breath, chestiness or tremors; Linden for fatigue, apathy, loss of appetite and to ease fears; Assam in the pause between trying to do ten jobs at once... this is a great reviver and especially liked by the older gentlemen who have appreciated having 'real' tea while serving abroad.,Camomile to soothe 'the wamblings of the stomach', this is especially good for abdominal migraine sufferers; Fennel takes a lot of beating as a soother for gall-bladder symptoms; China or Chrysanthemum is wonderful for easing neurasthenia and stress, while that good old standby Mint, is still one of the most reliable remedies for easing anything from headaches to heartaches! Do experiment with your teas and remember that, as you or your family probably drink more tea than anything else, you owe it to yourself and/or them to make your tea the best!

In Book One of this series I listed a veritable medicine-chest of remedies which could be simply made using just the herbs and spices most commonly used in the home, and if you have a real health problem, your remedy would probably be found in that volume. However, I will list a few herbal teas for you and, with some of these always to hand in the storecupboard, you will not only have a variety of flavours to titillate your taste buds, but also an ever present medicine supply for emergencies...

ANISEED... A champion remedy for any disease which creates breathlessness, including asthma, bronchitis, catarrh, etc.
BASIL.... The very best relaxant for the nervous system and one which eases anxiety, irritability, 'nerves', stress, P.M.T.
CINNAMON... No remedy is better than this for easing the pain of

flatulence, colic, biliousness and it clears diarrhoea too.
FENNEL.... A really pleasant taste makes this a must for anyone with dropsy, gall-bladder or kidney problems or obesity.
MARJORAM.... This is a real must for anyone with small children as it reduces fever, eases swollen joints and banishes grumps!
MINT..... One of the finest natural oxygenators known to man, this tea can be used as a pick-me-up, no matter what the problem is. It is tasty and equally as useful when taken either hot or cold, so should be in constant use in winter or summer for the relief of everything from acne to zits (I do believe that they are one and the same thing according to my son but I couldn't think of anything else starting with a ZED!), For a full list of the virtues of mint, I suggest you get Herb and Spice Remedies, and meanwhile, make sure you have some herb teas on your shelf.

There is however, one way in which the tea-bag can be of use...as a hot poultice to draw poisons out of boils, styes and whitlows: the high tannin content of a tea-bag make this an excellent and very effective remedy to keep at hand and,in the event of such a problem is simply solved by pouring hot water over the bag then applying it to the affected site while hot and keeping it there until it cools.After two or three applications of the same re-heated tea bag, the offending swelling will burst and the pain will leave as the matter clears. this is an excellent way to use your tea-bags!

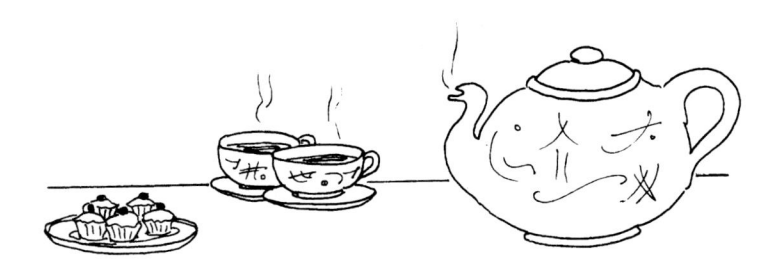

$\mathcal{V}$ is for Vinegar

Cider vinegar is the vinegar I would like you to have on the shelf of your new health-food medicinal store-cupboard. I cannot think of a more suitable food-medicine with which to end this little book as it is absolutely marvellous!
Anyone suffering from any of the following complaints would be well advised to throw out the acetic-acid-containing malt vinegar and replace it with Cider vinegar immediately:-

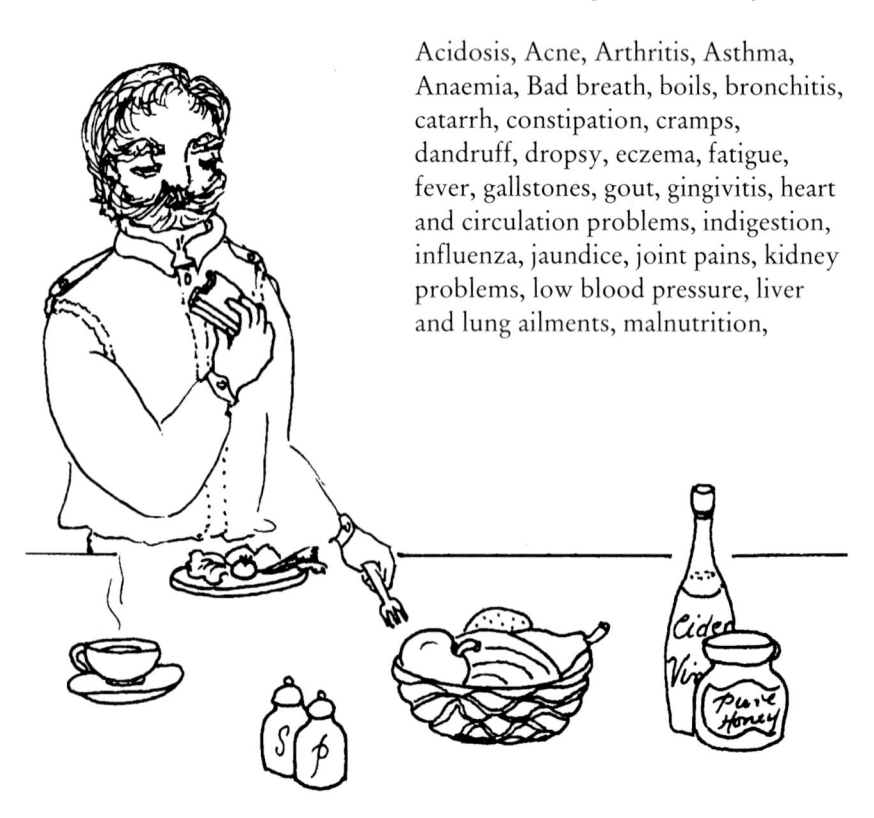

Acidosis, Acne, Arthritis, Asthma, Anaemia, Bad breath, boils, bronchitis, catarrh, constipation, cramps, dandruff, dropsy, eczema, fatigue, fever, gallstones, gout, gingivitis, heart and circulation problems, indigestion, influenza, jaundice, joint pains, kidney problems, low blood pressure, liver and lung ailments, malnutrition, muscle pain, nervousness, overweight, osteoporosis, pleurisy, pneumonia, quinsy, rheumatism, sinusitis, skin problems, stomach cramps, teeth and gum abscess, urinary disorders, weightloss and worms! Whew! What a remedy! As little and often is the best way to take Nature's remedies, all we really need to do is to take Cider Vinegar as our daily condiment, yet even for extreme cases taking the remedy is simplicity itself. All we have to do is to put one dessertspoonful of cider vinegar into a cup and fill the cup with hot water and take this as the first and last drink of the day, until we feel that it is no longer needed. For people with a sweet tooth, sweetening with honey to taste improves the taste and the efficacy of this wonderful medicine. Incredible!

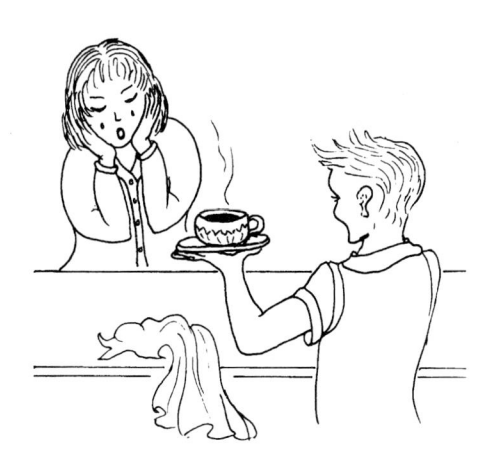

XYZ is for ...

There are many foods in the 'normal' store cupboard which we can still use in our new way of life so there is no need to despair over the precious time-saving cans and jars which are an absolute essential at times when it seems as if the whole population of the neighbourhood has arrived for a meal just when we have used the last of the fresh vegetables, the shops are shut and our reputation as a hostess is very much at stake!

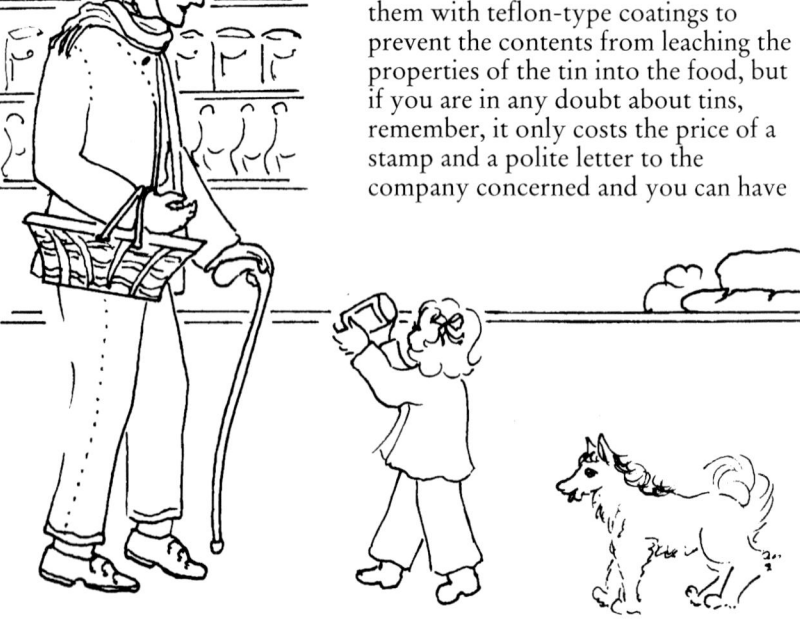

One thing which we must remember is that not all canners are as careful as others so always make sure that you 'go for gold' and accept no substitutes when the gold concerned is can-lining. Some manufacturers of cans also line them with teflon-type coatings to prevent the contents from leaching the properties of the tin into the food, but if you are in any doubt about tins, remember, it only costs the price of a stamp and a polite letter to the company concerned and you can have your assurance straight from the proverbial horse's mouth.

The old saying' you get what you pay for' is very true when it comes to canned goods and it is a false economy to buy cheaper brands as they contain poorer quality foods preserved with many chemicals and high amounts of toxic sugar. There are only a few good brands and they are household names and, being fully aware that the public are searching more now than ever before for good wholesome foods packed with the minimum of vitamin-loss, the packers of these products are improving their quality daily, so bearing this in mind, I am recommending you to use your cans.

There are just a few points which I would like you to bear in mind when buying cans for your store cupboard, and they will ensure that the convenience foods you have do not cause any inconvenience to your digestive system! Baked beans contain a high proportion of complex proteins and carbohydrates plus large amounts of valuable fibre and are one of the most valuable foods to have ready to eat in our health food store cupboard, but, be sure to buy only cans labelled 'no added sugar or salt' or 'low sugar' or 'no artificial colouring or preservative'. If you make sure of these points, the beans will contain many beneficial nutritives and be a health food! Red kidney, flageolet, black-eyed, butter, haricot, and many other kinds of canned beans contain many similar properties but all canned foods contain a little less goodness than do fresh. Sweetcorn or maize also contain a goodly amount of vitamins and minerals and, as detailed in the chapters on flours and grains, are very beneficial as body building foods, full of nutrition. Tomatoes are another very good taste-booster and quick snack to keep for emergencies, but, NOT TO BE TAKEN BY ARTHRITICS OR BY ANYONE SUFFERING FROM COLITIS OR ANY SIMILAR DIGESTIVE PROBLEM. Tinned fish is an excellent source of readily available protein but, when buying fish it is most important to remember that fish should always be packed in oil in order for it to give us the optimum nutrition (it also keeps for fives times as long when packed in oil as it does when packed in brine). The brine used to preserve fish in tins leaches into its flesh and can cause all sorts of fluid retention problems if eaten regularly.

While on the subject of fish, it is important to remember that fish oils are especially good and readily available source of Vitamins A and D, the sunshine vitamins, and we should all have plenty of fish throughout the winter in order to prevent us from getting the 'winter blues' (or, as they are now medically recognised and labelled, S.A.D.) Another benefit is, Arthritics, rheumatics and people suffering from osteoporosis will get especial benefit from taking fish in oil regularly. If you do not get enough sunshine or if you suffer from any of the preceding ailments, and cannot get fresh fish, it would be wise to include tinned fish fairly regularly in your diet.

Unlike fish, most tinned meats are loaded with preservatives and have no place on the shelves of our new optimum nutrition style store cupboards, so I am not listing any even as standbys. If good health is your first priority, you will not use them at all preferring instead fresh, farm fed meat from your local butcher. Many butchers now sell 'organic' meat, meaning that the animals have been fed on natural foodstuffs containing no chemical additives or hormones... watch for the sign and shop there.

While shopping, I always make sure that my stock of appetising taste-enhancers is kept replenished as, being both a person who enjoys good food and also a lazy cook, I often need something extra in a hurry so keep the following items in my cupboard.
Tomato puree, if it is packed using no additives, is a rich and tasty source of Magnesium which is an important aid to health for anyone suffering from High blood pressure, Kidney stones, Heart disease, Osteoporosis, and many stress-related illnesses including P.M.S. etc.... what an excellent way to take your medicine, simply by adding some tasty tomato puree to your cooking, this makes pastas, pizzas etc. into health foods! Garlic puree, paste, salt or granules are another marvellous 'quickie' to keep in your storecupboard and again, if processed properly contain so many nutrients to help strengthen every part of our bodies. I sometimes wonder how people manage without it. Anyone feeling 'under the weather' should try adding a little Garlic to their menu to pep them up, its magic! There is one important point about garlic that everyone should be aware of, GARLIC DESTROYS NEMATODES, and, if you eat deep sea fish or animal flesh (particularly pork) there is every chance that you may ingest these cold and heat resistant worms with your meals... but.. with garlic included in the meal they will be destroyed and harmlessly expelled. What a wonderworker! Horseradish sauce is another great taste booster which also helps our systems to digest the tough fibres of meats, cleaning stomach, intestine, colon and bowel in the process, also useful as a poultice to ease Arthritis. Horseradish is really a 'must'.

There are too many tinned, bottled and packaged foods available for me to list them all in this Little Book, but I hope that the advice which I have given you so far, will enable you to look carefully at the contents of these goods, I hope also to have given you a good idea of what to avoid and what can be utilised in your journey to good health via the shelves of your Store Cupboard.

Good Eating!
May you enjoy the rest of your life in vibrant Good Health.

Ailments and Remedies

The following pages have been produced to show a guide of those foodstuffs which are in the Store-cupboard..

You will be able to find the name of a common ailment on the left of the page and then search to the right to find the dot which corresponds to the page number indicated at the top of the page immediately below the name of that food item.
Select that food from the store-cupboard and then turn to the page indicated and read about the food and its qualities.

Please now turn this page over and find the food from the store-cupboard which will help to ease the ailments shown.

Headings	APPLE	BREAD	CEREALS	COFFEE	DRIED FRUIT	EGGS	FLOUR	GRAINS	HONEY	JAMS	KELP	LEMON	LENTILS
Page Number	8	11	15	19	22	27	30	34	36	41	43	45	49

Ailment

Ailment	APPLE	BREAD	CEREALS	COFFEE	DRIED FRUIT	EGGS	FLOUR	GRAINS	HONEY	JAMS	KELP	LEMON	LENTILS
Abscess					•				•				
Acidosis			•										
Anaemia	•		•	•					•				•
Appetite			•	•	•	•			•				•
Arteriosclerosis	•								•				
Arthritis	•		•						•			•	
Asthma	•				•				•			•	
Bad Breath									•				
Baldness									•				
Biliousness									•				
Bowels							•	•	•				
Bladder									•				
Blood							•		•				
Boils				•					•				
Bronchitis					•				•				
Cataracts	•								•				
Catarrh	•				•	•			•				
Circulation					•	•		•					
Colds					•	•			•				
Colitis	•				•		•		•				•
Conjunctivitis	•								•				
Constipation					•	•			•				
Cramps									•				
Coughs						•			•				
Dandruff	•								•				
Debility							•	•			•		
Diabetes	•		•				•	•			•		
Diarrhoea							•	•					
Dropsy									•				
Eczema					•				•			•	
Emaciation					•	•			•			•	
Emotions	•					•			•				

Headings	MOLASSES	NUTS	OIL	PASTA	PEPPER	RICE	SALT	SARDINES	SUGAR	TEA	VINEGAR	XYZ
Page Number	51	53	56	59	61	63	66	68	70	72	76	78

Ailment

Ailment	MOLASSES	NUTS	OIL	PASTA	PEPPER	RICE	SALT	SARDINES	SUGAR	TEA	VINEGAR	XYZ
Abscess											•	
Acidosis											•	
Anaemia											•	
Appetite			•						•			
Arteriosclerosis												
Arthritis				•		•					•	•
Asthma											•	
Bad Breath												
Baldness			•						•	•		
Biliousness												
Bowels												•
Bladder												
Blood												
Boils										•	•	
Bronchitis											•	
Cataracts												
Catarrh											•	
Circulation												
Colds										•		
Colitis												
Conjunctivitis												
Constipation			•	•					•			
Cramps				•					•			
Coughs				•		•					•	
Dandruff										•		
Debility												•
Diabetes												
Diarrhoea								•				
Dropsy												
Eczema												
Emaciation												
Emotions												

Headings	APPLE	BREAD	CEREALS	COFFEE	DRIED FRUIT	EGGS	FLOUR	GRAINS	HONEY	JAMS	KELP	LEMON	LENTILS
Page Number	8	11	15	19	22	27	30	34	36	41	43	45	49

Ailment

	APPLE	BREAD	CEREALS	COFFEE	DRIED FRUIT	EGGS	FLOUR	GRAINS	HONEY	JAMS	KELP	LEMON	LENTILS
Energy									•	•			•
Eyesight	•								•				
Fat													
Fatigue									•		•		•
Fertility									•				
Fever	•								•				
Grazes & Cuts	•								•			•	
Gallstones	•		•						•			•	
Gout	•			•	•				•				
Gums	•			•									
Hair							•		•				
Headache									•				
Heart								•	•				
Haemorrhoids					•				•				
High B.P.	•		•						•				
Hypoglycaemia								•	•				
Impotence									•		•		
Indigestion					•				•				
Infections									•				
Insect Bites	•						•		•			•	
Inflammation	•				•				•				
Insomnia	•			•				•	•				
Irritability								•	•				
Joints	•								•				
Kidneys	•			•					•		•		
Lip Sores									•				
Liver	•			•	•							•	
Low B.P.					•				•			•	•
Lungs	•								•				
Malnutrition									•				
Mental Depression									•				
Muscles	•						•	•					•

Ailment	Headings	MOLASSES	NUTS	OIL	PASTA	PEPPER	RICE	SALT	SARDINES	SUGAR	TEA	VINEGAR	XYZ
Page Number		51	53	56	59	61	63	66	68	70	72	76	78
Energy		•									•	•	
Eyesight			•										
Fat										•			
Fatigue		•					•				•	•	
Fertility													
Fever													
Grazes & Cuts										•			
Gallstones		•								•	•		
Gout		•				•				•			
Gums										•			
Hair										•			
Headache											•		
Heart										•	•	•	
Haemorrhoids													
High B.P.					•								•
Hypoglycaemia													
Impotence													
Indigestion					•						•		
Infections													
Insect Bites											•		
Inflammation													
Insomnia		•	•										
Irritability										•			
Joints					•					•	•		
Kidneys					•					•	•	•	
Lip Sores										•			
Liver										•	•		
Low B.P.										•			
Lungs										•			
Malnutrition		•								•			
Mental Depression					•						•		
Muscles					•						•	•	

Headings	APPLE	BREAD	CEREALS	COFFEE	DRIED FRUIT	EGGS	FLOUR	GRAINS	HONEY	JAMS	KELP	LEMON	LENTILS
Page Number	8	11	15	19	22	27	30	34	36	41	43	45	49

Ailment

Ailment	APPLE	BREAD	CEREALS	COFFEE	DRIED FRUIT	EGGS	FLOUR	GRAINS	HONEY	JAMS	KELP	LEMON	LENTILS
Nails	•					•	•		•				
Nappy Rash					•	•							
Nerves					•			•	•				•
Obesity	•		•						•				
Osteoporosis									•				
Pimples					•	•			•			•	
Pleurisy						•			•				
Rheumatism	•		•	•					•				•
Sinus									•				
Skin	•		•	•	•				•			•	
Stomach	•				•				•			•	
Stones									•			•	
Stress					•			•	•				
Styes	•								•				
Swelling Ankles					•				•				
Teeth	•					•			•			•	
Tongue	•								•				
Throat				•	•								•
Toxaemia						•			•				
Tonsillitis						•			•			•	
Syphilis					•				•				
Urinary	•								•			•	
Ulcers					•				•				•
Verruca									•			•	
Voice	•								•				
Vomiting									•				
Warts					•				•				
Water Retention									•				
Wamblings	•								•				
Weight					•	•			•		•		
Whitlows									•				
Worms			•	•	•	•			•				

86

Headings	MOLASSES	NUTS	OIL	PASTA	PEPPER	RICE	SALT	SARDINES	SUGAR	TEA	VINEGAR	XYZ
Page Number	51	53	56	59	61	63	66	68	70	72	76	78

Ailment

Ailment	MOLASSES	NUTS	OIL	PASTA	PEPPER	RICE	SALT	SARDINES	SUGAR	TEA	VINEGAR	XYZ
Nails	•											
Nappy Rash												
Nerves	•								•	•	•	
Obesity									•			
Osteoporosis								•		•	•	
Pimples												
Pleurisy									•			
Rheumatism	•								•			
Sinus									•			
Skin				•					•			
Stomach	•			•					•	•	•	
Stones												•
Stress									•		•	
Styes									•			
Swelling Ankles									•			
Teeth				•					•			
Tongue												
Throat										•		
Toxaemia												
Tonsillitis												
Syphilis												
Urinary									•			
Ulcers												
Verruca												
Voice												
Vomiting												
Warts					•							
Water Retention										•		
Wamblings										•		
Weight										•		
Whitlows										•		
Worms										•	•	

Notes